Take Control of
Type 1
Diabetes

A comprehensive guide to self-management and staying well

DR DAVID CAVAN

Vermilion
LONDON

1 3 5 7 9 10 8 6 4 2

Vermilion, an imprint of Ebury Publishing,
20 Vauxhall Bridge Road,
London SW1V 2SA

Vermilion is part of the Penguin Random House group of companies
whose addresses can be found at global.penguinrandomhouse.com

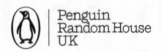
Penguin
Random House
UK

First published in the United Kingdom by Vermilion in 2018

www.penguin.co.uk

A CIP catalogue record for this book is available from the British Library

ISBN 9781785040931

Typeset in 11/17 pt ITC Galliard Std
by Integra Software Services Pvt. Ltd, Pondicherry

Printed and bound in Great Britain by Clays Ltd, St Ives PLC

Penguin Random House is committed to a sustainable future for
our business, our readers and our planet. This book is made
from Forest Stewardship Council® certified paper.

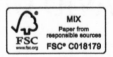

CONTENTS

FOREWORD

I have worked as a diabetes specialist for over twenty years. Very early on, I came to realise that the vast majority of diabetes management is done by the person with diabetes, and therefore it is essential that everyone with diabetes is given the appropriate training and education that will enable them to manage their diabetes as well as possible. From 1996 until 2013, I worked as a consultant at the Bournemouth Diabetes and Endocrine Centre. During that time I developed my interest in patient education, and in order to ensure people with type 1 diabetes had the appropriate skills to manage their diabetes effectively, in 1999 we launched a self-management programme for people with type 1 diabetes called BERTIE. BERTIE was quickly adopted by many other diabetes centres around the UK and many thousands of people with type 1 diabetes have attended courses based on BERTIE over the past fifteen years. However, aware that many people still did not have access to high quality self-management education, in 2005 we developed an online resource to teach the basics of carbohydrate counting and insulin dose adjustment. This has recently been updated and is available at www.bertieonline.org.uk.

There is a limit to the amount of information that can be provided in an education programme, whether 'face to face' or online and so I have written this book with the aim of providing a readily accessible and understandable resource that explains all aspects of the management of type 1 diabetes. My aim is that this book should provide very practical support to self-management. While the book is written for adults with type 1 diabetes, many aspects will be relevant to older teenagers. I am not a children's diabetes specialist and the book does not cover the management of type 1 diabetes in younger teenagers or children. While some parts of the book may be of interest to the parents of children with type 1 diabetes, I would recommend the following books that specifically address the needs of children and their parents:

▶ *Type 1 Diabetes in children, Adolescents and Young Adults*, by Dr Ragnar Hanas, a paediatric diabetes specialist from Sweden provides a huge amount of information relevant for the parents of a small baby with type 1 diabetes, right through to the needs of young adults.

▶ *Help, My Child has Type 1 Diabetes*, by Roxana Reynolds, who herself has type 1 diabetes, provides advice, information and real stories for parents and carers of a child with type 1 diabetes.

Take Control of Type 1 Diabetes has been written to support people who have just been diagnosed with type 1 diabetes, right through to those that have had the condition for many years. Although there has been a big expansion in availability of patient education in the past fifteen years, it is sadly the case that many people diagnosed before 2000, in the UK at least, received very little education on how to manage their type 1 diabetes. Very often, those who did receive education did so by attending a single course, perhaps many years ago. It is my hope that this book can help all people with type 1 diabetes fill the gaps in their knowledge about the modern management of type 1 diabetes.

The management of type 1 diabetes is entering a very exciting phase, with new insulins and technologies becoming available that have the potential to revolutionise the management of type 1 diabetes. Thus I have aimed to cover the latest developments in insulin pump therapy, continuous glucose monitoring and new insulins that provide great hope for the future. Even with these advances, it is still the case that the person with type 1 diabetes will need to take into account the impact of their lifestyle, physical activity and their food choices on their blood glucose control, and so the book provides extensive details about these aspects.

Since the early years of this century, the focus of much teaching has been to encourage people with type 1 diabetes to eat what they like, in the belief that the modern insulins now available would be able to cope with all types of diet. My experience in the years since then, has led me to the firm belief that this is not always true. Not even the best available insulins and technologies can manage meals with very high sugar or starch content and keep blood glucose within the normal range at all times. In the past several years, therefore, I have encouraged patients with type 1 diabetes to restrict their carbohydrate intake as an important means of achieving good control of their glucose levels, and the rationale for this is discussed in the book.

The book has been written primarily for a UK audience; however in order to make it relevant to readers elsewhere, the book includes sections for those for whom the insulins commonly in use in the UK are either not available or affordable. Blood glucose measurements are provided in mmol/l (as used in the UK) as well as in mg/dl (as used in US and many other countries).

1

THERE IS ALWAYS HOPE

Living with type 1 diabetes is not easy. It often develops in children or young people who are very healthy, and then suddenly they have diabetes. It also frequently starts at a time of life where being different is a big deal. It always demands attention be given to food, activity levels and many other day-to-day occurrences that otherwise would not require such consideration. It requires regular injections of insulin and blood glucose checks. It can spring surprises for no obvious reason. It can be physically, emotionally and psychologically draining. It can lead to nasty health problems down the line. It is always there.

These are just some of the truths about living with type 1 diabetes. It is not surprising that all too often, a person with the condition can feel overwhelmed, out of control and worried about their present or future health – or just burnt out. Yet staying healthy demands that a person with type 1 diabetes cannot afford to let such feelings dominate and impact upon their ability to manage their diabetes.

If you or someone close to you has type 1 diabetes, this book has been written for you. My hope and aim is that it will be of support in providing you with the knowledge, skills and tools you need to take control of the diabetes. It is natural to experience concern or worry, but my hope is that in the following chapters you will find practical guidance on how to overcome some of the challenges your diabetes might pose.

I do not have type 1 diabetes, so I cannot claim to have the personal experience of someone that does. However, over more than twenty years I have had direct experience in supporting people with type 1 diabetes, from the time of diagnosis right through to those who have had the condition for decades – including many who remain very healthy. As you will read, I was moved by the problems I saw in those whose diabetes was not well controlled, often through no fault of their own, and determined in my own way to improve the support and education available. This book is my attempt to make that experience available as widely as possible.

The book has been written particularly to support those at the time of diagnosis. The reason for this is that it is well recognised that things that happen around that time – both good and bad – can have a long-lasting effect. So the better you can deal with the diagnosis, the quicker you can take control of your diabetes, and the sooner you can deal with any negative issues surrounding diagnosis – the better the outlook for the future.

If you have recently developed type 1 diabetes, how does this make you feel? Before doing anything else, it is worth pausing to consider this, in order to address any feelings that might get in the way of being able to take control of the condition in the future. People experience a whole range of feelings when they are diagnosed with type 1 diabetes, from relief that they know what was causing troublesome symptoms or anger that it should affect them, to fear for the future, loneliness and a whole host of other feelings and emotions. Such responses are completely natural, and it is good to acknowledge them and if possible to talk about them with someone close to you who is able to listen, even if they don't have the answers to the many questions you may have.

The reason for discussing this right at the beginning is because if certain emotions are not properly addressed, they can have a massive effect on your physical health, as well as mental health, for years to come. There are a number of helpful and supportive websites, which include discussion forums where you can share your feelings with others who have been through the same experience, which I recommend you look at. Some of these are listed in Appendix 1 (see page 329).

However, whatever your own situation, I encourage you not to worry. Our understanding of type 1 diabetes, and our ability to control it, has changed beyond all recognition over the past twenty years, and we are learning more all the time. As a result of these advances, the risk of disabling complications has reduced significantly. In addition, there are now education programmes available in many parts of the country and online, where you can learn how to take control of your diabetes and protect your long-term health.

The message of this first chapter is 'there is always hope'. These were the words of comfort I gratefully received from a caring nurse where my father was admitted on Christmas Eve in 2012. He had been diagnosed with chronic lymphocytic leukaemia. This is a relatively common condition in the elderly and generally does not cause serious health problems. Unfortunately, he had a rare and aggressive form of the condition that did not respond to standard treatment. His specialist explained to us that there was a different treatment that he could have, that it was complex and had significant side-effects but it had a chance of taming his disease. I could tell from the tone of the doctor's voice that it was serious and that the chances of success were slim. However, I was struck by the focus on the possibility of a positive outcome. And that positivity had a deep and encouraging effect on my father, as well as our family around him.

The day after he was admitted, on Christmas day, I was struck by how ill he looked and I was extremely worried. One of the nurses could see that in my face, and she said to me, very gently and very kindly those four words: 'There is always hope.'

That focus on the positive, on hope, was a great source of strength. Arguably the hope for a person with type 1 diabetes is so much greater, especially with recent advances in management and technology available, yet often I meet people with type 1 diabetes who seem devoid of hope, as well as some diabetes professionals who focus more on the perceived negatives of having type 1 diabetes than on the positive hope for the future. And so, whether you or someone you love has just been diagnosed with type 1 diabetes, or whether you have had it for many years, my aim is that the information provided in this book will give you a greater sense of hope. There is much about type 1 diabetes that can seem difficult and unfair. Yet, as I have experienced over the past twenty-five years in working with and helping those with type 1 diabetes, there is so much that can be done to make life easier.

So, what are your hopes in respect of your type 1 diabetes? As you read this book, it will be helpful to have set out your goals in doing so. That will help you focus on the areas that are most important to you. I encourage you to think about – and write down – the answers to the following questions. And if you are not really sure just yet, that is fine – I will remind you again later.

- What are your reasons for reading this book?
- What frustrates you most about having diabetes?
- How do you want things to be different?

- How will you know when you have achieved this?
- What is the main thing you would like to change after reading this book?

We will look at your answers to these questions in chapter 22.

My hope is that the information in this book will provide reassurance and hope for the future.

2

WHAT IS TYPE 1 DIABETES?

A HISTORY OF DIABETES

The full name of the condition is diabetes mellitus, which literally means 'passing [perhaps more accurately "pissing"] honey', as in diabetes the urine contains glucose and so tastes sweet. Diabetes was described in ancient Egypt, in the Papyrus Ebers, which dates from around 1500BC, as a disease where urine is too plentiful. Sushruta of the Hindus wrote in 1000BC that the urine was sweet and that ants and flies were attracted to it. He thought that diabetes was a disease of the urinary tract (kidneys and bladder) and wrote that it could be inherited or develop as a result of dietary excess or obesity (perhaps referring to type 1 and type 2 diabetes). The recommended treatment was exercise. It was not until the seventeenth century that it was discovered that the urine was sweet because it contained sugar and that diabetes was a disease of the pancreas rather than the kidneys. This was established in 1682 by

Johann Brunner, who removed the pancreas from dogs and found this led to diabetes. In 1797, John Rollo, the surgeon-general of the Royal Artillery, wrote a book in which he described the case of a Captain Meredith, who took a diet low in carbohydrate and high in fat and protein. His weight fell from 105kg to 73kg (or 230 to 160lb) and the symptoms resolved.[1] At that stage diabetes was reported as being relatively rare, and associated with wealth.

It was not until the end of the nineteenth century that the role of insulin became apparent. In 1889 Mehring and Minkowski removed the pancreas from dogs to cause diabetes. This was then reversed by transplantation of small pieces back into the peritoneum (the lining of the abdominal cavity).[2] In 1921 Banting and Best isolated an extract of pancreatic islet cells and found this reduced glucose levels in diabetic dogs.[3] The following year, this extract (a prototype of insulin) was injected for the first time into a patient with diabetes, a 14-year-old boy called Leonard Thompson.

Piece by piece the puzzle was being completed, such that by the 1920s, it was established that diabetes is characterised by an excess of sugar (glucose) in the blood, causing excess in the urine. The disease was often seen in overweight people, in whom it could be controlled by adopting a low carbohydrate diet. In other patients, insulin, extracted from animal pancreases and given by injection, led to a fall in blood glucose levels.

TYPES OF DIABETES

By the 1970s, it had become clear that there are two distinct types of diabetes:

1. Type 1 diabetes usually first occurs in children or young adults. It comes on quite suddenly with marked symptoms such as thirst and weight loss, and can only be treated with insulin.

2. Type 2 diabetes usually occurs in later life, and it has become increasingly clear that it is related to increasing weight gain, as a result of excess food intake and/or too little exercise. Its onset is often much more gradual without causing any specific symptoms, and it is sometimes diagnosed by a screening blood test. Type 2 diabetes can be controlled by lifestyle changes, principally by modifying diet. Many people are prescribed drugs to control type 2 diabetes, and until relatively recently it was thought that most people would eventually need insulin.

Since then our understanding has developed further, inasmuch as there are rare forms of diabetes that occur in young people (so called maturity-onset diabetes of the young or MODY). These are inherited conditions, are not associated with weight gain, and there is usually a strong family history of diabetes. Although they usually present in childhood, most cases can be controlled with tablets rather than insulin.

It has also become apparent that the distinction between type 1 and type 2 diabetes is not as clear cut as previously thought, and for those who are diagnosed in the forties and fifties, there may be a period of uncertainty before one can definitely distinguish between the two. For example, some overweight adults present quite acutely with very high glucose levels and require insulin at diagnosis, but can later be switched to tablets. Conversely, there is a type of type 1 diabetes that occurs in older people, sometimes referred to as latent autoimmune diabetes of adulthood (LADA). Like type 1 diabetes, people with this condition are not overweight; however, the onset is more like type 2 diabetes, and they may be treated with tablets for a period. Within a few years, it becomes clear they need insulin, and from that time behave very much like type 1 diabetes.

Gestational diabetes is a condition in which diabetes occurs during pregnancy. It is similar to type 2 diabetes and can be controlled with diet in some cases, otherwise insulin is used, as tablets are generally not advised in pregnancy. It usually reverses once the baby is born, but both the mother and the child are at increased risk of developing type 2 diabetes in later life.

Diabetes can also arise as a result of other diseases affecting hormones (e.g. acromegaly, caused by too much growth hormone, or Cushing's disease, caused by too much cortisol). These cases generally reverse once the underlying condition has been treated. Cortisol is the body's natural steroid, and people who have been treated with steroids for long periods of time for conditions such as asthma may develop diabetes. Diabetes also occurs if the pancreas is affected by other diseases, or if the pancreas has been wholly or partly removed.

MAKING A DIAGNOSIS OF DIABETES

The typical symptoms of diabetes include excessive urination, excessive thirst, tiredness, blurred vision, weight loss and infections such as thrush. These arise because in diabetes, glucose cannot enter the body's cells and so it accumulates in the blood stream. As glucose is not getting into the body's cells, these are starved of energy leading to weight loss and tiredness. As the blood glucose rises, the kidneys try and excrete the excess glucose in the urine. This explains why glucose can be detected in the urine, causing infections such as urine infections and thrush. In order to excrete glucose, the kidneys need to emit a larger volume of water (otherwise you would pee out sugar lumps), and this leads to dehydration. In turn this prompts excessive thirst, and high glucose levels in the eyes lead to blurred vision.

In many cases of type 1 diabetes, especially in children or young adults, the onset of symptoms is quite rapid and diagnosis can easily be made by measuring the blood glucose level. The symptoms of type 1 diabetes can deteriorate rapidly, leading to a condition known as diabetic ketoacidosis due to lack of insulin. This can lead to coma and even death if insulin treatment is not started, and is discussed in more detail in chapter 5.

Type 1 diabetes can also be mistaken for other conditions, especially in parts of the world where it is quite rare, and in some countries medical staff may make a mistaken diagnosis of malaria, TB or even HIV in young children with diabetes. Even in countries such as the UK, where type 1 diabetes is relatively common (although still much less common than type 2 diabetes), early symptoms may be missed, leading to uncontrolled high glucose levels and the development of ketoacidosis. Especially in those diagnosed in their thirties or above, type 1 diabetes is often of slower onset and with much milder symptoms causing an initial diagnosis of type 2 diabetes as described above.

Diabetes is diagnosed by blood tests. This means that if you have symptoms which you think may be due to diabetes but the blood tests are normal, you do not have diabetes. On the other hand, if your blood tests are diagnostic of diabetes, then you have diabetes even if you do not have any symptoms. The tests that are used to diagnose diabetes are either a measurement of random blood glucose, a fasting blood glucose test, a glucose tolerance test or by a glycated haemoglobin test.

With type 1 diabetes, the rapid onset usually means that the random glucose level is high enough to make a diagnosis of diabetes, and it is rarely necessary to use one of the other diagnostic tests.

1. Random blood glucose

This is often the first test that will be done. It is taken at any time of the day after breakfast. The results are expressed as the amount of glucose molecules per litre of blood (mmol/l) in the UK or as the weight of glucose per decilitre of blood (mg/dl) as used in the US, Germany and many other countries. They are interpreted as follows:

Random blood glucose level	Interpretation
Up to 7.7mmol/l (139mg/dl)	Normal
7.8 to 11.1mmol/l (140–200mg/dl)	Impaired glucose tolerance
Above 11.1mmol/l (200mg/dl)	Diabetes

If the random glucose is normal it is unlikely that the person has diabetes; however, if it is within the impaired glucose tolerance range, then a fasting glucose or a glucose tolerance test will usually be performed, as described below. Impaired glucose tolerance and impaired fasting hyperglycaemia (see below) describe an intermediate state, sometimes known as 'pre-diabetes', that identifies people at risk of developing type 2 diabetes. It is rarely relevant in the diagnosis of type 1 diabetes.

2. Fasting blood glucose

This is a blood test taken after a fast of 12 hours, during which time only water can be taken by mouth. It is generally taken first thing in the morning. The results are expressed as the amount of glucose molecules per litre of blood and interpreted as follows:

Fasting blood glucose level	Interpretation
Up to 6.0mmol/l (109mg/dl)	Normal
6.1 to 7.0mmol/l (110 to 126mg/dl)	Impaired fasting hyperglycaemia
Above 7.0mmol/l (126mg/dl)	Diabetes

If both the fasting and random glucose levels are normal, then the diagnosis is not diabetes.

3. Glucose tolerance test

This is a standardised test where a fasting glucose level is measured, and then the patient is asked to drink a liquid that contains 75 grams of glucose. A further blood test is taken two hours after the drink to see how high the glucose level has risen. The results are interpreted in the same way as the fasting and random tests above. If either the fasting OR the two-hour values are diagnostic, then the patient has diabetes. Both have to be normal to exclude the diagnosis.

4. Glycated haemoglobin (HbA1c)

When the level of blood glucose is higher than normal, the excess glucose attaches to a number of different molecules in the body. (So, for example, glucose attaching to the lens in the eye can lead to cataracts developing, or attaching to soft tissue in the shoulder can lead to frozen shoulder.) This is termed glycation. Red blood cells contain haemoglobin. This is the substance that carries oxygen in the blood cells, to take to the different tissues around the body (and which gives blood its red colour). A small amount of haemoglobin is glycated, and how much depends on the amount of glucose in the bloodstream. Red blood cells last for about 4 months before they are 'recycled', and the amount of glycated haemoglobin in any one cell gradually increases over this time. Blood glucose levels change constantly according to food intake and activity levels, and so a single measurement is of little use in monitoring diabetic control. Glycated haemoglobin (abbreviated as HbA1c), on the other hand, is used to assess glucose levels over a longer period of time, and for many years has been the gold standard means of assessing diabetic control. In 2009 it was also introduced as a means of diagnosing diabetes.

Historically, HbA1c was expressed as the percentage of haemoglobin that was glycated. In 2011, a new system of units was introduced, which expresses the glycated component as a concentration of the total haemoglobin (mmol/mol). It was intended that this system should be adopted globally, however, old habits die hard, and many countries, and much international literature, still use the old system. I will therefore present both units in this book. In people without diabetes, glycated haemoglobin is generally below 40mmol/mol (5.8 per cent). A measurement of 48mmol/mol (6.5 per cent) or above is considered diagnostic of diabetes. However, it is important to be aware that a level below this does not rule out diabetes, and if there is any doubt then a glucose tolerance test should be performed.

THE ROLE OF INSULIN IN KEEPING GLUCOSE LEVELS UNDER CONTROL

In order to understand why glucose levels rise in people with diabetes, it is important to understand how insulin controls glucose levels when everything is working normally.

Glucose is a type of sugar which is used by nearly all cells in the body for energy. It is essential that all parts of the body have a steady supply of glucose. This glucose is obtained from the food we eat: all carbohydrates (sugars and starch) that we eat are broken down into glucose, which is then absorbed from the gut into the bloodstream, so that it can be carried to all tissues and used as energy. Any spare glucose is taken up into the muscles and liver where it is stored in the form of glycogen. Glycogen in the muscles is then available for later use if the muscles need extra energy (for example, during intensive exercise). Once the glycogen stores are full, excess glucose is converted to fat and stored in the liver.

While glucose only enters the body when we eat or drink, the body's cells require a constant supply of glucose to function properly. This is provided by the liver, which releases some of its stored glucose into the bloodstream to ensure that just the right amount is available during periods when we are not eating – for example, overnight. In a person without diabetes, the amount of glucose in the bloodstream is kept at around 4–6mmol per litre (70–110mg/dl).

The level of glucose in the bloodstream is controlled by insulin, a hormone produced by the pancreas. The pancreas is an organ which sits just below the rib cage, behind the stomach. Like many of the body's organs, the pancreas does lots of different things. However, it has two main functions. One is to produce enzymes, which are released directly into the small intestine to break down food so it can be absorbed into the bloodstream. These enzymes include amylase, which breaks down starch into glucose; lipase, which breaks down fat; and protease, which breaks down proteins.

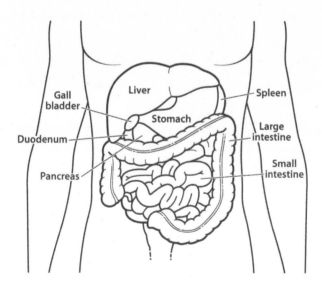

The other main function of the pancreas is to produce hormones. These are chemicals which are released into the bloodstream and have effects all around the body. Insulin is one of the hormones produced by the pancreas, and its job is to regulate the amount of glucose in the bloodstream to ensure that cells get the right amount of glucose at all times. Insulin is produced by specialised cells, known as beta cells, which are found located in clumps of cells scattered throughout the pancreas and known as the Islets of Langerhans, or islets for short. Insulin acts in the following ways:

1. When we eat a meal, the carbohydrate in the meal is converted into glucose in the gut and passes through the gut wall into the bloodstream. The body detects that the glucose level in the blood is rising and this leads to the pancreas producing additional insulin.
2. The insulin acts on individual cells to allow glucose to enter them. Insulin molecules attach to a receptor on the cell membrane, which opens up to allow glucose in. This is often compared to insulin being like a 'key', which opens the 'door' for glucose to enter the cell.
3. The insulin also stops the liver and the muscles from releasing stored glucose into the blood; this allows spare glucose to be added to the glycogen stores.
4. When we are not eating, the pancreas produces a continuous small amount of insulin to control the release of glucose from the liver. In the liver, insulin is like a tap, which turns off the release of glucose from the liver. If glucose levels in the blood drop too low, then less insulin will be produced (opening the tap), allowing more glucose to be released from the liver. On the other hand, if glucose levels rise, then more insulin is produced, closing the tap and slowing down the release of glucose from the liver.

In type 1 diabetes, the body stops producing insulin as a result of the body's immune system destroying the insulin-producing beta cells in the pancreas. This means there is no insulin to turn off the tap releasing glucose stored in the liver into the bloodstream, or to open the doors to allow glucose to enter body cells after a meal.

As a result, glucose accumulates in the blood and rapidly rises to high levels. In type 1 diabetes, treatment with insulin rapidly restores glucose levels to normal.

This is in contrast to the situation in type 2 diabetes, where the body produces insulin but it doesn't work very well. It seems that the problem starts in the liver, which becomes 'immune' or resistant to the effect of insulin, so that even if insulin is present, the liver just keeps releasing glucose into the blood stream. This is called 'insulin resistance' and to try and get around this, the pancreas produces more and more insulin in an attempt to control the release of glucose from the liver. Therefore, treatment with insulin is rarely as effective as with type 1 diabetes. For a while this may work in keeping the blood glucose level under control, but eventually the liver becomes resistant to even these high levels of insulin, and the level of glucose in the blood rises high enough to make the diagnosis of diabetes.

Type 2 diabetes is increasing rapidly across the world, and is associated with modern day lifestyles characterised by unhealthy diets (especially of processed foods high in sugar, salt and unhealthy fats), lack of physical activity and increased body weight. People with type 2 diabetes are often perceived as being in some way to blame for their condition; while there is undoubtedly an element of choice in what we eat and what we do, the big rise in type 2 diabetes has resulted from significant changes to our food, and our physical and work environments, that are often not in the control of any one individual. Such stigmatisation is thus inappropriate.

It is even more unfortunate that many members of the general public (and even some health professionals) fail to distinguish between type 1 and type 2 diabetes and apply the same stigma to people with type 1 diabetes. It is thus easy to understand why some with type 1 diabetes would prefer it had a different name to avoid this confusion.

THE BLURRED BOUNDARY BETWEEN TYPE 1 AND TYPE 2 DIABETES

Earlier in this chapter we learnt that the distinction between type 1 and type 2 diabetes is not as clear-cut as was once thought, and several different 'types' of type 2 diabetes have now been identified. The diagnosis of type 1 or type 2 diabetes is usually done clinically, that is according to the symptoms and signs present at the time of diagnosis rather than by any formal testing. The reason for this is that there is no readily available test that will say for definite whether a person has type 1 or type 2 diabetes. The nearest we have are tests to check the levels of different antibodies to the islet cells that are present in many, but not all, people with type 1 diabetes. If these antibodies are present in the bloodstream it is very likely the person has type 1 diabetes. However, if they are not found, the individual may still have type 1 diabetes.

The other test that can be performed is to check the level of c-peptide in the blood. C-peptide is a by-product of the production of insulin, and for every molecule of insulin produced in the pancreas, one molecule of c-peptide is also produced. It is uncertain whether c-peptide has any biological effect, but it is very useful as a marker of insulin production. So, if it is found in the blood, it means that insulin is definitely being produced and the person is therefore likely to have type 2 diabetes. This information has to be used with caution as many people with type 1 diabetes continue to produce insulin for up to two years (during the honeymoon period as explained starting on page 109), and there is now evidence that some insulin production may last for up to five years.)

There is also the matter of ketones: ketones are substances found in the blood that result from the breakdown of fat. When the body cannot produce the insulin required to enable glucose to be used by the body's cells for energy, then fat is broken down for the necessary energy instead, and this in turn produces ketones. At high levels ketones can cause the blood to become acidic, and this is the basis of the condition known as diabetic ketoacidosis (DKA). Ketones can be tested for in the blood using a special meter and test strips, similar to those used to test blood glucose. Alternatively, a urine test (using a ketone test strip) can be performed to check for evidence of ketone production. A small amount of ketones will be present in the urine of someone who has not eaten for several hours, but higher levels of ketones in someone with diabetes generally mean that they are deficient in insulin, and need insulin treatment.

It was generally thought that if a person had ketones in their urine (or blood) at the time they were diagnosed with diabetes it meant they had type 1 diabetes. They would then be started on insulin and told they would need insulin treatment for life. Over recent years, however, it has become apparent that some people labelled, in all good faith, as having type 1 diabetes, do not actually have it. When tested they have c-peptide in their blood, demonstrating that they are producing insulin, and, in some cases it has been possible for them to stop insulin treatment altogether.

While some parts of this book may be helpful to people with other types of diabetes, it is intended specifically to help people with type 1 diabetes learn how to manage their condition. The rest of this book refers solely to type 1 diabetes.

WHAT CAUSES TYPE 1 DIABETES?

The relatively easy part of the answer to this question is that type 1 diabetes results from the destruction of the beta cells in the pancreas.

To recap, the pancreas is a very interesting organ that sits just behind the stomach. It has two distinct functions. The first is to produce enzymes that are released into the gut to digest food. The second function is to produce hormones. These are chemicals that are released into the bloodstream and exert their action on cells in different parts of the body, as with the example of insulin.

The hormone-producing cells are found in small clumps of cells called the Islets of Langerhans, which are dispersed through the pancreas. The insulin-producing cells are called beta cells. However, the islets contain a number of different cells that produce other hormones. The main one relevant to people with diabetes is glucagon, which is produced by the alpha cells. Glucagon has effects that are the opposite to insulin, including raising blood glucose levels if they fall too low. It is available as an emergency treatment to treat hypoglycaemia, or dangerously low blood glucose levels. Other types of islet cell include delta cells that produce somatostatin (a hormone involved in the regulation of the production of insulin and glucagon) and gamma cells that produce pancreatic polypeptide (which regulates the production of stomach and pancreatic enzymes that digest food).

In type 1 diabetes, the beta cells are destroyed as a result of attack by the body's immune system. Interestingly, the other islet cells continue to function normally, although over time alpha cell function can become impaired, leading to reduced secretion of glucagon. Quite why the immune system singles out the beta cells for attack remains much of a mystery, despite years of research to try and find the answer. What is known is that type 1 diabetes results from a combination of having the right (or wrong) types of genes that prime the immune system to attack the beta cells, and exposure to something in the environment that acts as the trigger to launch the attack.

The genes that predispose to type 1 diabetes

I am often asked whether type 1 diabetes is hereditary, and the answer is not entirely straightforward. From the above, it is clear that our genes play a role and as these are inherited from our parents, then this part of the risk of developing type 1 diabetes is indeed hereditary. However, diabetes only develops after the immune attack has been triggered, and the trigger is almost certainly something in the environment, such as a virus for example. Thus type 1 diabetes is not a true hereditary disease such as cystic fibrosis, which is always present in a child who inherits the affected gene from both parents. However, a child of a mother who has type 1 diabetes has a 3 per cent risk of developing it; this compares to a 5 per cent risk in a child whose father has type 1 diabetes and an 8 per cent risk in a child whose brother or sister has it.[4] This is much greater than the 0.1 per cent risk in a child who has no immediate family members affected and shows the influence of genes in increasing the risk of developing type 1 diabetes. However, it is still a relatively low risk, underlining that while genes play a role, there is something else that triggers the onset of type 1 diabetes.

For many years, it has been known that certain genes are associated with an increased risk of developing type 1 diabetes. The strongest associations are with so-called HLA genes that regulate the immune system. Many years ago, in the early 1990s, I spent three years working in a laboratory as part of a team that was trying to pinpoint which of these genes were most closely linked to type 1 diabetes and why. I learnt many things in that time. I learnt that there were many different genes associated with type 1 diabetes, and that these associations were different in different races. I also learnt that laboratory scientists have to work extremely precisely for their experiments to be successful; and as a result of many unsuccessful experiments, I realised I was not really suited to a life working in a laboratory. Twenty-five years later, automated machines now undertake many of the procedures that relied on my (lack of) precision and our understanding of the detail of these genetic influences has increased exponentially. But we are still far from knowing all the answers about how and why certain genes increase the risk of type 1 diabetes. So, what do we now know?

Perhaps the strongest associations are with the HLA genes known as DR3 and DR4; individuals who have one of these two genes are at increased risk of type 1 diabetes; those that possess both are at an even greater risk. On the other hand, the gene DR2 appears to protect from type 1 diabetes (although it is associated with other autoimmune conditions such as multiple sclerosis).

Earlier in this chapter I mentioned that certain antibodies are present in many people with type 1 diabetes, especially before or around the time of diagnosis. The commonest antibodies are to insulin itself, known as insulin antibodies, and antibodies to the enzyme called glutamic acid decarboxylase (GAD). GAD is an enzyme involved in the production of GABA, a chemical used to transmit signals between nerve cells in the brain (a neurotransmitter). It appears that GAD is also produced in the islet cells, which provides a possible link with type 1 diabetes. It is now recognised that people with different HLA genes tend to have different antibodies: those with HLA DR3 tend to produce GAD antibodies, initially at least, whereas individuals with DR4 tend to produce insulin antibodies first.

Antibodies are molecules produced by the immune system to react with or bind other molecules and facilitate their destruction by specialised immune cells. These associations suggest that the genes related to type 1 diabetes are therefore in some way associated with the immune attack that eventually leads to beta cell destruction. However, the situation is much more complex than just the few genes we have discussed so far as over 50 distinct genes have been identified that influence the risk of developing type 1 diabetes.

The trigger for the immune attack

The first part of the puzzle of what causes type 1 diabetes is the genetic make-up, which increases the likelihood of the immune system attacking the islet cells. The second part of the puzzle is the trigger that sets off the immune attack. The fact that the numbers of new cases of type 1 diabetes are increasing in many parts of the world suggests that something within the environment has changed to trigger these new cases (as our genetic makeup will not have changed that much to cause the increase).

We have discussed how the appearance of antibodies provides evidence of the immune attack against the beta cells. These antibodies generally appear in early childhood, in toddlers between the ages of one and two, although type 1 diabetes may not actually occur until some years later. By studying children known to have these antibodies, researchers have identified a number of possible triggers that set off the immune attack. These possible triggers, or environmental risk factors, include viral infections, particular foods in the diet and toxins. The strongest link with viruses is with enteroviruses. These are viruses found in the gut – one of the most well-known is the polio virus, others cause symptoms of the common cold or can lead to meningitis. One theory is that an enterovirus infection during pregnancy is associated with a later immune attack in the child to cause type 1 diabetes. Some studies have suggested that frequent respiratory infections in the first six months of life could also be associated with an increased risk of type 1 diabetes.[5]

Some studies showed that breastfeeding protects from type 1 diabetes and it has been suggested that early intake of cow's milk could increase the risk of type 1 diabetes in children. A small study showed that babies who received cow's milk had double the risk of developing islet cell antibodies later in childhood compared to babies who did not. However, it has not been shown conclusively that this led to increased development of type 1 diabetes.[6]

Type 1 diabetes is more common in areas that are further from the equator. Therefore, rates are higher in Scandinavia and Australia than, for example, in Africa.[7] One explanation for this finding is that low levels of vitamin D increase the risk of developing type 1 diabetes. Vitamin D has many important functions, relating to bone strength and also in regulating the immune system. The body can make vitamin D, but adequate exposure to sunlight is necessary to produce sufficient amounts. As sunlight decreases with increasing distance from the equator, then populations living in colder climates have lower vitamin D levels – and higher rates of type 1 diabetes. Paradoxically, in the far north of Norway, there is less type 1 diabetes than further south, despite there being very little sunlight to make vitamin D during winter. However, in these areas, there is a high intake of fish in the diet, and fish oil is a rich source of vitamin D. A number of studies have shown that providing vitamin D supplements in childhood does protect against the development of type 1 diabetes.[8]

The final possible type of trigger is so-called beta cell stress. It has been suggested that a number of factors that increase the need for insulin to be secreted could place too heavy a demand on the beta cells that then become stressed. Such factors include being overweight, puberty, infections and trauma. Major life events (such as a death in the family) and other psychological traumas lead to increased stress hormones such as cortisol, that also cause beta cell stress. Regardless of the cause, it has been suggested that excessive demands on the beta cells can prompt a reaction of events within the cells triggering the autoimmune process that leads to type 1 diabetes.

So how do we put all this together? It is evident that there are still a number of possible theories about what causes type 1 diabetes, and it is likely that the precise cause is different in different people. We can say with some degree of certainty that certain people are at increased risk of developing type 1 diabetes because of their genes. However, having these genes in itself is not sufficient – there also needs to be the right combination of environmental factors in early life. Two of the most likely culprits are early exposure to cow's milk and low vitamin D levels. (This is remarkably similar to the situation in multiple sclerosis, another autoimmune disease that affects the nervous system.) Finally, in those with the right genes and the right environmental factors, there is often an acute event, such as an infection, that leads to the disease showing itself. From this, it will be clear that type 1 diabetes is not primarily determined by any specific behaviours by the person who develops type 1 diabetes.

3

BASIC PRINCIPLES OF TYPE 1 DIABETES TREATMENT

Having read the previous chapter, you will hopefully have a reasonable understanding about the metabolic abnormalities that are present in type 1 diabetes. The following chapters will provide greater detail about the complexities of managing type 1 diabetes (and as I said right at the beginning, the successful management of type 1 diabetes is not easy, and it can be very complex). The aim of this chapter is to provide a broad overview of the principles of treatment. These principles will underpin the approach recommended in the rest of the book.

THE FIRST PRINCIPLE – THINK LIKE A PANCREAS

In the last chapter, we discussed how type 1 diabetes results from an immune attack on the beta cells that produce insulin. Although some insulin production can continue for a few of years after diagnosis (the so-called 'honeymoon period'), at the end of the day, the impact of type 1 diabetes is a complete lack of the hormone insulin. And so the main focus of the treatment of type 1 diabetes is to replace insulin as closely as possible to how the pancreas secretes insulin naturally. Indeed, one of the best-known books that promotes this principle is called *Think Like a Pancreas*.[9] And 'thinking like a pancreas' is a good place to start. Unlike type 2 diabetes, type 1 diabetes is not a condition related to unhealthy lifestyles, obesity or excess liver fat causing problems with insulin resistance. A person just diagnosed with type 1 diabetes is usually young, fit and healthy, but with a pancreas that no longer produces insulin. So, the principle is to replace the lacking hormone, just as those whose thyroid gland no longer works have to take tablets to replace the missing thyroid hormone, or those whose adrenal glands no longer work take tablets to replace the missing cortisol.

Although the management of type 1 diabetes is based on the replacement of insulin, it is much more complex than the management of almost all other hormone deficiencies. Apart from replacing the missing insulin, it also requires regular measurement of the level of glucose in the blood and modifications to diet that recognise that the lack of insulin means that the body is less able to manage certain foods, particularly those that are high in carbohydrates.

It is also more complex in that the pancreas normally secretes a low amount of insulin continuously (called basal insulin) and then produces rapid spikes or boluses of insulin when glucose levels rise, for example after eating a meal. Replacing insulin to mimic a fully working pancreas therefore requires what is known as a 'basal bolus regimen', to reflect the two types of normal insulin secretion.

The basal insulin is the background insulin that is injected every day (usually once or twice daily), regardless of any food eaten. Traditional basal insulins include NPH or isophane insulin, such as

Insulatard™ or Humulin I™. More recently, long-acting analogue insulins have been developed that are absorbed more smoothly than traditional insulins. For many with type 1 diabetes, use of a long-acting insulin analogue appears to provide more stable glucose control, with less hypoglycaemia, particularly at night. The most commonly used analogues are glargine (Lantus™) or detemir (Levemir™). It is important to establish the correct dose of basal insulin that will keep blood glucose levels stable (if no food is eaten), so that it does the same as the pancreas would do if it were working normally.

The bolus insulin is the insulin that is injected before each meal. Previously, soluble insulin was used as the bolus insulin (for example Actrapid™ or Humulin S™, or Humulin R™ in the US). Many people with type 1 diabetes now use rapid-acting analogues that have been modified so that they are absorbed much more rapidly. These are associated with less hypoglycaemia between meals. Commonly used analogues include lispro (Humalog™), aspart (Novorapid™ or Novolog™) and glulisine (Apidra™). It is important that the dose of each bolus is adjusted according to the carbohydrate content of the meal to be taken, with adjustments made according to anticipated activity levels and to whether the current blood glucose level is too low or too high (which I explain in full in Chapters 12 to 17).

Thus an effective regimen that replaces insulin as closely as possible to the human pancreas will usually require one or two injections of basal insulin and at least three injections of bolus insulin every day. If an insulin pump is used, a continuous infusion of rapid-acting insulin provides the basal cover, with bolus delivered manually via the pump as required. Other insulin regimens include twice-daily injections of basal insulin or of a mixture of basal and bolus insulin. However, these do not mimic the pancreas as closely as the basal bolus regimen. They also place quite rigid restrictions on the timing and quantity of meals, as their dose cannot easily be altered on a day to day basis.

THE SECOND PRINCIPLE – THE AIM OF TREATMENT IS TO MAINTAIN NEAR-NORMAL BLOOD GLUCOSE LEVELS

Insulin does many useful things in the body but as far as type 1 diabetes is concerned, the most important is to keep the level of blood glucose as near-normal as possible. That will ensure that you avoid glucose levels that are dangerously low or high, which can both cause immediate and unpleasant symptoms and potentially lead to a medical emergency. It will also ensure than in the longer term, your diabetes does not cause damage to various parts of your body as a result of high glucose levels. So, what does that mean in practice?

First, it is important to understand what is meant by 'normal' blood glucose levels. The 2015 UK Guidance from the National Institute of Health and Clinical Excellence (NICE) on management of type 1 diabetes[10] states that glucose levels should aim to be:

- Between 5 and 7mmol/l (90–126mg/dl) first thing in the morning (fasting);
- Between 4 and 7 mmol/l (72–126mg/dl) before meals and at other times of the day;
- Between 5 and 9 mmol/l (90–162mg/dl) at least 90 minutes after meals.

The guidance also states that people with type 1 diabetes should be supported to maintain their HbA1c level at 48mmol/l (6.5 per cent) or lower.

Now, if you have been recently diagnosed your levels will probably be much higher than that. That is fine, but the aim should be to gradually work towards these levels for good long-term health.

Maintaining this level of glucose control is not easy and requires regular measurement of glucose levels. This is done using a commercially available meter and test strips. As a minimum, it is recommended that the glucose level is checked before each meal and before bedtime. Glucose should also be checked before every insulin injection; if feeling unwell; before, during and after exercise; and before driving. NICE recommends that up to 10 tests a day may be necessary.

In the UK, meters are generally available free of charge from diabetes clinics, and the strips needed to make measurements are available free on prescription. In this regard, we are very fortunate, as in many other countries, part of the cost has to be paid for by the person with diabetes. In some of the poorest countries, the whole cost has to be borne by the individual, and when the cost of insulin is also taken into account, paying for treatment can often take up a very large portion of their total income.

THE THIRD PRINCIPLE – FOUR IS THE FLOOR

An important aim of treatment is that one's blood glucose level should never drop below 4mmol/l (or 70mg/dl). This is because any blood glucose level below this level risks falling further and leading to hypoglycaemia. Once the glucose level is below 3mmol/l (54mg/dl), there will not be enough glucose available for the brain and other organs to function properly. This causes a number of symptoms that result from the effect of hormones such as adrenaline (causing tremor, sweating, hunger) as it tries to counter the effect of insulin and increase the glucose levels. Other symptoms (such as drowsiness and confusion) result from the brain being starved of glucose. Unless corrected by taking in glucose, the blood glucose level can fall further to cause fits, coma and even death. It is essential that you are able to recognise the early warning symptoms and act to prevent a dangerous hypo.

You will notice that the 'floor' has been set at 4, which is a little higher than the level normally associated with hypoglycaemia. This is to provide a 'safety buffer' to allow for the fact that insulin treatment is not an exact science and blood glucose meters are not always 100 per cent accurate.

This is very important, as if the glucose level drops to 3 or below on a regular basis, the body adapts by losing the warning symptoms of hypoglycaemia. It is as if it accepts low glucose values as the 'new normal', and therefore decides there is no need to react with symptoms. This is called hypoglycaemic unawareness and means that a person can be running along with a glucose level of less than 2mmol/l (36mg/dl) and still feel they are functioning normally. Yet their brain is being starved and they are at risk of becoming unconscious with no warning. It used to be thought that hypoglycaemic unawareness was a permanent feature that happened in people who have had type 1 diabetes for many years. However, it is now known that if a person with hypoglycaemic unawareness can avoid hypoglycaemia (by making four the floor) then their symptoms will return and they again become aware of hypoglycaemia. So the principle of 'four is the floor' is extremely important. It also means that if you are experiencing both low and high glucose levels, it is important to work on preventing the lows as a priority. Very often then the highs will sort themselves out, as will be discussed further in chapters 7–11.

THE FOURTH PRINCIPLE – LOW CARBOHYDRATE FOODS MAKE IT EASIER TO ACHIEVE NORMAL GLUCOSE LEVELS

The aim of treatment is to keep glucose levels as normal as possible. As almost every meal will lead to an increase in glucose levels, then it makes sense to try and make life a bit easier for you (and for your insulin) by avoiding consuming large quantities of carbohydrates – the vast majority of which are turned into glucose by the body's digestive system. Although modern insulins are very good, even 'rapid-acting' insulins do not work as quickly or as effectively as naturally-produced insulin. There was a vogue about ten years ago to think that a person with type 1 diabetes could eat anything they wanted, as long as they took the correct insulin dose. The years of experience since then have convinced me that this is just not true. I therefore recommend that you recognise the limitations of injected insulin: even a large dose simply cannot keep up with very large amounts of carbohydrate. There is some evidence that a high dose of rapid-acting insulin is not quite as rapid as a lower dose, and also risks bringing the glucose level too low and causing hypoglycaemia.

The traditional diet recommended for those with diabetes (and everyone else for that matter) is one that is based on starchy foods.[11] As all starch is turned by the body into glucose, that advice has never seemed very logical to me for the treatment of diabetes. Friends of mine with type 1 diabetes tell me they restrict their carbohydrates if they want to achieve the best control they can and I firmly believe that the standard advice is potentially detrimental to people with any type of diabetes. I cannot think of a single other condition, which is exacerbated by a certain type of food, where the recommended diet is to base all meals on exactly the foods that exacerbate it. So my very basic diet plan, which I will discuss in much more detail in chapter 12 (see page 163), is as follows, with the aim of trying as a rule to have no more than 25–30g with each meal:

	Yes	No
Breakfast	• Eggs, vegetables • plain yoghurt (not low fat), with berries/seeds/nuts	• Cereals • Toast • Fruit juice
Lunch	• Soup (not root veg) • Salad	• Sandwiches • Crisps/chips
Evening meal	• Meat, fish, chicken • Lots of green veg • No or small portion only of starchy carbohydrate	• Rice-, potato- or pasta-based meals
Snacks	• 1 small piece of fruit • Handful of nuts • Small piece of cheese • Hard-boiled egg	• Biscuits, cookies, cakes, sweets/candy • Dried fruit

In recent years, there has been a lot of debate about which foods are best for us, whether fats really do make us fat and whether carbs are really that good. Things are changing, but only slowly. The official Diabetes UK advice is no longer to base all meals on starchy carbohydrate, and their most recent report on diet acknowledges that carbohydrates have the greatest influence on blood glucose levels,[12] yet many of their recipes are heavy in carbohydrate, and they still recommend 150ml of fruit juice as being an appropriate food choice – even though, with 12–15g of fast-acting sugar, it will cause a rapid rise in blood glucose level.

THE FIFTH PRINCIPLE – JUST ABOUT EVERYTHING YOU DO AFFECTS BLOOD GLUCOSE LEVELS

I have heard it said so often that a person with type 1 diabetes can do anything, it just requires a bit of adjustment. While the first part is undoubtedly true, the second is in my opinion a massive understatement. The reason is that, if you have type 1 diabetes, just about everything you do affects your blood glucose level. There are the obvious things like eating – most foods will have some effect on increasing blood glucose levels; alcohol – which can decrease or increase glucose levels depending on its relative content of alcohol and carbohydrate; and exercise – which will often reduce the blood glucose level (unless it is anaerobic exercise which usually increases it). Then there are the less obvious, like routine physical activity, such as housework, shopping, walking the dog or sexual intercourse, all of which can cause the blood glucose level to drop, sometimes quite sharply. Or stress, which often causes an increase in the glucose level, but sometimes can cause a decrease. Illness can cause quite a significant increase in glucose levels, even in the context of a minor illness such as a cold. And if that isn't enough, women have the added issue of the menstrual cycle, which in some people can be associated with very troublesome fluctuations in glucose level, as a result of the impact of changing hormone levels on the effect of insulin. And there are probably many more that I am not even aware of.

In writing this, my aim is not to overwhelm you with thinking that achieving stable glucose control is an impossible task, because it isn't. But it does require a lot of learning basic information about how insulin works, about how your body responds to different foods and different situations, and about what you can do to ensure you have good glucose control as much of the time as possible.

THE SIXTH PRINCIPLE - EDUCATION IS ESSENTIAL FOR GOOD MANAGEMENT OF TYPE 1 DIABETES

Whether you are reading this book as a person with type 1 diabetes, or for someone close to you, you have to live with the condition for 8,760 hours every year (8,784 in leap years). You may spend less than two hours a year with a health professional to discuss diabetes. That leaves 8,758 hours (or 99.9 per cent of the time) when you have to manage the diabetes yourself. And as I have illustrated, unlike other hormone problems, it is not just a question of taking a tablet or an injection every day, it requires a more detailed level of understanding of the principles of diabetes management than most doctors and nurses have. It also requires the ability to solve problems independently, as for most of the time, you will know far more about your diabetes than anyone else you are in contact with.

I have had the privilege of helping many thousands of people manage their type 1 diabetes over the past 25 years. Some of my earliest experiences had a big impact on me, as they revealed just how unprepared I was to provide meaningful advice. Early in my career, I recall a man who was in his late twenties. He was married with young children and worked in a factory. His life was overwhelmed by glucose levels that fluctuated wildly, from very low to very high levels, and he was at a complete loss as to how to escape this vicious cycle that was completely dominating his existence and impacting on his family life and his work. The tragedy is that I and the other members of the team were pretty clueless about what to do as well, as in the early 1990s there was very little training in the UK of either health professionals or people with diabetes on the practicalities of managing type 1 diabetes. My role in the diabetes clinic was generally to advise a small increase or decrease in insulin dose to people who were usually on two injections a day, and thus with little hope of successfully managing all the influences of daily life on their glucose levels. And those were the days before the Internet, which nowadays at least enables people who find little joy from their diabetes clinic to have a wealth of support and resources available to help them.

That man's plight has stayed in my mind ever since. Those early experiences led me to realise that not only did I need to up my game in diabetes management, but all health professionals needed to ensure that people with type 1 diabetes and their carers were provided with education so that they had the knowledge and the skills necessary to manage the condition. It led me some years later to work with the diabetes team in Bournemouth in developing what I called an 'Educational Model of Care', which simply means that education of the person with diabetes (or the carers responsible for them) to manage their condition has to be at the foremost of everything we do.

This emphasis on education led first to the development of the BERTIE course in 1999. BERTIE is a course that consists of four day-long sessions at weekly intervals, to train people with type 1 diabetes in key self-management skills, with a focus on carbohydrate counting and insulin dose adjustment (see chapter 11). This was followed by the development of a structured educational approach to the management of the first year with type 1 diabetes ('Living with Diabetes') in 2004, to an online carbohydrate counting course in 2005 (recently updated as BERTIEonline[13]) and to a structured educational model of care for insulin pump therapy in 2010. And it has led to this book, which aims to provide you with all the information needed to make a success of managing type 1 diabetes. Of course, a book cannot replace the input from a skilled educator, nor the benefits of a group education course, but I hope it can act as a resource when those other elements are not available.

This sixth principle builds upon the other five and emphasises the primary importance of self-management education to everyone with type 1 diabetes. And it is never too late to learn. I can think of many, many people who lived with type 1 diabetes for several years, experiencing debilitating fluctuations in their glucose control, who benefitted enormously in later life from attending a BERTIE course where they learnt some basic principles on how to match their insulin to their food intake and their activity levels.

4

DIABETIC KETOACIDOSIS (DKA)

For some people, diabetic ketoacidosis is part of the experience of being newly diagnosed with type 1 diabetes. For others, it is unfortunately a regular feature of their life with diabetes. While some episodes of DKA might not be preventable, the vast majority are. A key aspect of successful self-management of type 1 diabetes is to avoid DKA as far as possible and that is why I feel it deserves a chapter all to itself.

So, what is diabetic ketoacidosis? It is, as the name suggests, a condition in which the blood becomes acidic as a result of having a very high concentration of ketones (the chemicals released when fat is converted to energy instead of glucose). There is also a high concentration of glucose in the blood, together with a high potassium level and dehydration that is often quite severe. All these changes result from a lack of insulin, as follows:

1. <u>High blood glucose</u>: We have already discussed the importance of insulin in regulating the concentration of glucose in the blood. In a person without diabetes, a lack of insulin is generally a sign of fasting or starvation, and so when insulin is not present, the body responds with the release of glucose from the glycogen stores in the liver. With the complete absence of insulin, as is often the case in DKA, this release is uncontrolled, and rather than comparing the release of glucose from the liver to a leaking tap, as described previously, in DKA it is more like a burst water main. This is in addition to any glucose absorbed from the gut remaining in the blood. The body also responds to the lack of insulin (that it mistakes for starvation) by breaking down protein in order to produce more glucose and releasing it into the bloodstream. This is a process known as gluconeogenesis (literally: production of new glucose). The combined effect of these processes is to cause high, and sometimes very high blood glucose levels. The highest I have seen is just over 100mmol/l (1800mg/dl) in a person with severe DKA. On the other hand, it is possible to have DKA with only mildly elevated glucose levels, and so these cannot be used to judge the seriousness of the condition.

2. <u>Dehydration:</u> This arises from the high blood glucose level. In an attempt to reduce it, the kidneys excrete glucose into the urine and that also requires them to excrete large volumes of water. Hence frequent urination is a common symptom in someone with high glucose levels. In addition, vomiting is very common in DKA and this can worsen dehydration significantly. Severe dehydration, with loss of fluid from cells, increases the risk of drowsiness and possible coma.

3. <u>High blood ketone levels (ketosis):</u> Just as a lack of insulin leads to the production and release of glucose into the bloodstream, it also leads to the breakdown of fat stores in the

liver. These are in the form of fatty acids that are converted to three molecules known as ketones (acetoacetate, beta-hydroxybutyrate and acetone). These enter the circulation and are taken up by cells to be used as energy (they cannot use the glucose in the blood as most cells require insulin to enable it to enter the cells). As with the release of glucose from the liver, release of ketones is essentially uncontrolled when no insulin is present. Ketones are also released as a by-product of gluconeogenesis, the production of new glucose described above.

4. Excess acidity of the blood (acidosis): The two main ketones (acetoacetate and beta-hydroxybutyrate) are acidic and as their concentrations rise, the blood becomes increasingly acidic. Acidity is measured by pH, and the lower the pH, the more acidic the blood. The normal pH of blood is 7.4, and so as ketone levels rise, the pH falls progressively. In DKA the pH is usually less than 7.3; in severe DKA, the pH can be less than 7.

5. High potassium level in the blood: Insulin controls many biochemical processes and one of these is the transport of potassium into cells. In DKA, the lack of insulin can cause a significant loss of potassium from the body's cells into the blood, leading to high blood potassium levels. This is also exacerbated by the acidosis. This in itself can be dangerous as a high potassium level can cause heart rhythm disturbances.

You will see from the above that DKA can cause multiple disturbances of normal metabolism, and can lead to coma, heart rhythm problems and, if left untreated, will eventually be fatal. This is why it is so important that a person with type 1 diabetes understands the seriousness of DKA, and knows how to detect its early warning signs. These will be discussed in more detail in chapter 7, but for now it is important that any time you feel unwell and your glucose level is above 14mmol/l (250mg/dl), you should check the ketone levels in your blood or urine, monitor your glucose frequently and be prepared to inject extra insulin. If you start to vomit or become drowsy, you should be taken immediately to a local Emergency Department for assessment and possible admission.

DKA is clearly bad news. The good news, however, is that all of these metabolic abnormalities can be readily reversed by rehydration and treatment with insulin. In DKA, fluids and insulin are both given via a drip directly into a vein. However, each disturbance has the potential to cause problems, and constant monitoring is essential to keep track not only of the blood glucose level, but also the potassium level and pH as well as pulse, heart rhythm and blood pressure. In order to measure the pH, a blood sample needs to be taken from the brachial artery in the wrist. This can be quite uncomfortable and, in my experience, is one of the things many people particularly dislike about having type 1 diabetes. It is also important to monitor urine output and so in many cases, it is recommended that a urinary catheter is inserted. As DKA is often associated with vomiting, a tube may need to be inserted through the nose into the stomach. This is both for comfort and to avoid the risk of choking on any vomited fluid. For this reason, most guidelines recommend that the initial management of DKA should take place in a high dependency or intensive care unit.

The other good news about DKA is that it is relatively rare. The most recent national audit in UK suggests that only around 4 per cent of people with type 1 diabetes experience DKA in any year.[14] As stated earlier, with ready access to high quality insulin and monitoring equipment, most cases of DKA can be prevented and I hope that the information contained in this book will help you minimise the risk of ever developing it. The situation is very different in those parts of the world where insulin is either unaffordable or simply not available.

As a result, in some countries, running out of insulin is sadly still a common cause of DKA and death, even nearly 100 years after the first use of insulin as a treatment for diabetes.

It is important not to confuse DKA with the state of ketosis or ketogenic diets. Ketosis describes the situation where the body uses fat for energy, and has been promoted as an efficient means of losing weight, and in some cases to reverse type 2 diabetes. It is achieved by having a very low carbohydrate intake, so that the body switches to using fat stores for fuel. It is the basis of the Atkins diet. The big difference from DKA is that in a state of ketosis induced by such a diet, insulin is still being produced and glucose levels are normal and thus the drastic metabolic changes seen in DKA do not occur. Despite this, I have heard professionals, including those working in diabetes, appear to confuse ketosis with DKA. It is important not to confuse the two, as some people with type 1 diabetes use a ketogenic diet with good results. We will discuss this in more detail in chapter 12.

5

INITIAL MANAGEMENT OF TYPE 1 DIABETES

THE PRESENTING SYMPTOMS OF TYPE 1 DIABETES

The classic symptoms of type 1 diabetes are thirst, passing excess urine and weight loss. Especially in children and young adults, these can arise very rapidly and become very marked, with extreme thirst and weight loss developing over a few days. The most vivid description of this came from someone who posted their experience at diagnosis on the forerunner of the BERTIEonline website. The person recalled that as a young child, they were unable to reach the tap to get a drink of water and so sucked on the wet flannel that was on the edge of the basin. These symptoms arise from the high level of glucose in the blood, leading to glucose being excreted together with high volumes of water, in the urine. The glucose in the urine is also a breeding ground for bugs, and it is not unusual that this often leads to thrush in both men and women. High glucose levels in the eye can make it difficult to focus and so blurred vision often accompanies these symptoms.

If someone recognises these symptoms as being suggestive of diabetes, then a quick finger-prick blood test, or a urine test will be enough to confirm the suspicion and allow immediate treatment to be instigated. If the symptoms are not recognised as being due to diabetes, and this still occurs all too often, then the person's condition will deteriorate until they develop ketoacidosis. In this case, urgent hospital admission is required in order to correct the metabolic derangements as described in the previous chapter.

For older adults, the presentation is not quite so acute, and rather than developing over a few days, symptoms can come on more gradually over a period of weeks and even months. This can be associated with other symptoms that result from the effect of prolonged high glucose levels on various tissues, in particular the nervous system. These can include tingling or pins and needles, due to the irritation of nerve endings by high glucose levels, and also erectile dysfunction, again through an effect of high glucose on the nerves.

As the prime abnormality in type 1 diabetes is deficiency of insulin, then the priority is to start insulin treatment as soon as possible. Unless a person is in ketoacidosis, this does not usually require hospital admission in the case of adults, but often it is customary to admit children to initiate treatment for type 1 diabetes. However, it is important that they are seen the same day and that they are diagnosed by someone with expertise in managing diabetes. In the UK, this generally means a visit to the local specialist diabetes centre.

For someone recently diagnosed, I think it could be helpful to set out what I consider the essential steps in the initial management.

THE FIRST DAY: CONFIRMING THE DIAGNOSIS – PERFORMING A BLOOD TEST

The first thing that will be done is to take some details of the symptoms experienced and a blood finger-prick test to check the blood glucose level. This will confirm the diagnosis of diabetes (if it is above 11.1mmol/l or 200mg/dl) and help determine the initial insulin dose that will be required. It also provides an opportunity to learn how to check one's own blood glucose – as this will be an essential part of the management of type 1 diabetes for the future. This involves using a finger-prick device to draw a small drop of blood from the finger that is placed onto a test strip. You then insert the strip into a meter that after just a few seconds provides an accurate reading of the glucose level. There are a number of different meters available and it is not within the scope of this book to explain the precise instructions for each of them. However, it is essential that the person demonstrating blood-testing technique is fully conversant with the meter that is being used, and is able to explain the procedure in detail.

In addition to glucose, a blood sample can be sent off to measure the initial HbA1c, as this will be important in assessing progress over the longer term. A blood or urine test for ketones will help confirm the diagnosis is type 1 diabetes (although ketones can also be found in some with newly diagnosed type 2 diabetes). If there is any doubt (typically in middle-age adults) then a blood sample can be taken to measure the antibodies and c-peptide, as discussed in chapter 2 (see page 18).

In the case of young children, the first few days following diagnosis will take place in hospital so that you and they can feel supported and reassured.

The first insulin injection

The immediate need is to start insulin. Some years ago, there was a vogue to start people initially on a twice-daily insulin mixture (of fast-acting and intermediate acting insulin). The aim was usually to switch to a multiple injection basal bolus regimen, however in my experience, this change was never seen through in many cases. Perhaps because of what has become known as 'clinical inertia', sometimes through a rather judgemental attitude as to whether an individual could cope with four or more injections a day, and sometimes because the team actually didn't feel it was of any benefit. And then there is the understandable view of many patients, who perceived a switch from two to four injections as representing more intensive treatment and meaning their condition had worsened, and who shied away from making the change. Whatever the reason, it struck me that if a basal bolus regimen is the ideal treatment for type 1 diabetes, then each person deserved to be provided with it from day one.

However, when I was working in Bournemouth in the late 1990s, the initial insulin treatment was determined to a very large extent by which doctor was available in the department to write the prescription. So, one of my first actions in developing a uniform model of care for type 1 diabetes was to stipulate that everyone would indeed start on a basal bolus regimen. In the UK, we now have NICE guidelines that recommend this, and so I hope that this 'insulin lottery' is now very much a thing of the past.

Of course, one of the great advantages of the basal bolus regimen is that it encourages us 'to think like a pancreas', and immediately instils in each person with newly diagnosed type 1 diabetes the understanding that there is a requirement for basal or background insulin 24 hours a day, and then boluses to cover each meal.

When it comes to the bolus (mealtime) insulin, there are currently three choices that are all very similar to each other. These are the rapid-acting analogues lispro (Humalog™), aspart (Novorapid™ or Novolog™) and glulisine (Apidra™), and I do not recommend any one over the other. They should be given just before eating a meal. In areas where these are not available, soluble insulin can be used, for example Actrapid™ or Humulin S™ (or Humulin R™ in the US). Ideally, these need to be given at least 30 minutes before eating, in order to have the optimal effect.

So on day one, it is essential that anyone newly diagnosed with type 1 diabetes is taught how to give themselves an injection, and ideally gives it there and then.

Then to the injection itself. In the UK, the majority of insulins are available in cartridges to be used with injection pen devices, so there is no longer any need to use a needle and syringe to draw up the correct dose, rather the user dials up the dose on the insulin pen, and then injects. In some other countries, such as the US, injection pens are often quite expensive and so needles and syringes are still used quite commonly. As with blood glucose meters, each insulin has its own pen, and they all differ in some ways and it is not in the scope of the book to cover the detail of how to use each once. Again, it is essential that the person demonstrating injection technique is fully conversant with the pen that is being used, and is able to explain the procedure in detail. Giving the first injection is an important milestone for anyone when first diagnosed. Many people have quite understandable expectations that the injection will be difficult or painful, and many are very pleasantly surprised, relieved and encouraged both at how short and fine the needle is (4–6mm or ⅕in) and how painless the injection is.

There are a number of different areas in the body where insulin can be injected. The main thing is to inject into fat below the skin. Most people have sufficient fat for this purpose in the upper arm, abdomen, thigh or buttocks. I generally recommend injecting mealtime (bolus) insulin into the abdomen, within 10cm (4in) of the umbilicus.

Basal insulin can be injected into the thigh. It is important, right from the start, to get into the habit of rotating injection sites. This means injecting into a different spot, but within the same area of the body, each time. So, if you inject three mealtime boluses each day, the first can be above and right of the umbilicus, the second below and right, the third below and left, and so on. The same with the basal injections in the thigh, maybe upper right thigh on one day, upper left the next day, then lower right, then lower left. Changing sites each time makes it less likely that insulin will build up in the fat in any one place. If it does so, then it will cause that area of tissue to grow and become thickened, which then makes it more difficult for the insulin to get into the bloodstream.

At this early stage, one would generally be advised to take a fixed dose (that is, the same dose) of bolus insulin with each meal, as the aim is gradually to bring glucose levels down, rather than fine tune each dose (as will be covered in detail in chapter 11).

When the fast-acting insulins were first introduced, it was suggested that they could be given after a meal. I strongly advise against this, as by the time an after-meal injection has reached the bloodstream, the glucose absorbed from the meal could already have caused the blood glucose level to reach quite a high level. There are some situations, such as eating out, when you might not know exactly how much insulin you will need to take. In this situation, I generally advise to take a dose before you eat, and if necessary top it up with an extra dose afterwards. They key is that there should already be some insulin in your system once the glucose from the meal hits your bloodstream. Therefore, in an ideal world, the dose should be given at least 15 minutes before you eat, although in practice this may not always be possible.

Now for many years, the basal insulin has been a single injection at bedtime, initially of intermediate-acting insulin and for the past several years, of a long-acting analogue such as glargine (Lantus™). The second long-acting analogue to be made available, detemir (Levemir™), is not quite so long acting, and ideally should be given twice a day, although many people only take it once a day. In 2015, NICE recommended that twice-daily detemir should be the first-choice basal insulin; however, for many people (those with diabetes and their healthcare advisors) this is possibly an injection too far, especially right at the beginning. When long-acting analogues are not available, traditional basal insulins such as NPH or isophane insulin (such as Insulatard™ or Humulin I™) can be used. It is possible for the first basal insulin injection to be given during the clinic visit; otherwise it should be given that evening at home. Again, the need at this early stage is to bring glucose levels down gradually, and depending on the response, the dose will need to be reviewed every few days. In young children, the dose may need to be adjusted every day, usually during the stay in hospital.

Information about diabetes and diet changes

Day one isn't the time to go into a lot of detail about diabetes and diet, but the profound thirst can lead people to drink excessive quantities of sugary drinks that of course just make the glucose level even higher. Thus, it is important to avoid high sugar foods and drinks completely and to particularly use water to quench the thirst. It is also important to understand that symptoms will disappear rapidly once insulin has been started, and that over the coming weeks and months, all necessary information and education will be provided to help you master management of type 1 diabetes.

THE FIRST WEEK

Over the first week, it is important that you are reviewed frequently to assess glucose levels and use these to determine if and how insulin doses should be adjusted. If glucose levels are coming down rapidly, then it will be necessary to reduce insulin doses. On the other hand, if they are not budging, or only very slowly, then some doses may need to be increased. Where necessary, blood testing and insulin injection technique should also be reviewed.

Ideally an appointment with a dietitian will take place to introduce the concept of carbohydrate counting. The first step of this is to explain which foods contain carbohydrate and how to assess their effect on blood glucose levels.

THE FIRST MONTH

This will also be the time when more detailed information about diabetes and diet changes can be given, as well as starting the process of teaching how to adjust insulin doses, how to manage hypos and how to cope with illness – so-called 'sick day rules'. During this period, people are usually feeling pretty much back to normal and so issues such as return to work (if applicable) and driving can be discussed. They are also coping with injections and blood tests, and often managing to maintain stable glucose levels, and all appears well.

And then they fall into a black hole.

Or, rather, that was the case in many clinics where I worked, where having reached this stage, an appointment is given to come back to the clinic in about six months and meanwhile the person is asked to call the clinic should he or she run into any problems. But what constitutes a problem? How will they know whether it is a problem that requires review? What if insulin requirements change? And what if … ?

THE FIRST YEAR

Unfortunately, the answers to the 'what if' questions very much depended on the individual and how they responded to the challenges that inevitably come along during the first few months of living with type 1 diabetes. Some people head straight back to their clinic for advice, some muddle on and work through and succeed. Others, through muddling on, adopt self-management (or 'survival') practices that either constrain their lifestyle and/or lead to high glucose levels, perhaps in response to a bad hypo.

To address this, when we set up the BERTIE programme nearly 20 years ago, we suggested that those with newly diagnosed diabetes should attend a structured education programme around six months after diagnosis. This was in contrast to the standard advice at other centres, which was to wait until two years after diagnosis. Two years seemed a very long time in which people can learn self-management behaviours that are not ideal, and the longer those behaviours have become routine, the harder it can be to change them. So we decided on six months. However, we soon found that even this was too late for some people, who had struggled since they had been left to fend for themselves, feeling unsupported. We also noted that many were in the honeymoon period, when their insulin requirements were very low indeed, and could suddenly increase at any time, meaning more re-learning will be needed. In this respect, a longer wait could be justified.

So, what had become the 'gold standard' of diabetes education – a structured education programme – didn't seem to be right for people in the first year of type 1 diabetes. Joan Everett, one of the diabetes nurse specialists in Bournemouth (who had done much of the ground work in setting up the BERTIE programme), set out to find a solution. In 2003, she gave a presentation at the International Diabetes Federation's Diabetes Congress in Paris, on our experience in setting up BERTIE. At that congress, she came across a presentation from a team in Cuba that had developed an approach to the education of people with type 1 diabetes. This involved a group education session every three months from the time of diagnosis, that replaced traditional clinic visits – and it seemed to work. We therefore set about replicating this, and the first 'Living with Diabetes' session took place in January 2004.

THE 'LIVING WITH DIABETES' PROGRAMME

The principle behind 'Living with Diabetes' or LWD for short was very simple. On the first Wednesday of every third month (January, April, July and October), we invited everyone that had been diagnosed with type 1 diabetes during the previous 12 months to come together for the morning. Following diagnosis, people received individual advice from the team, as described above, for the first month and during the second month following diagnosis had an appointment with a consultant to review progress and to arrange any further tests that might be necessary if there was any doubt about the diagnosis, or concern about how things were progressing. All being well, an appointment was then made for the next LWD session; I explained that this is how we would provide the care needed for the first year. This was because, from previous experience, if we put on these sessions as an 'optional extra', some people would choose not to attend. We even made the appointment letters look like a clinic appointment letter (this also meant that the hospital got paid a fee which enabled us to run the sessions without getting into trouble from the managers). And so, at each LWD session, a group of up to 15 people would gather. Some would have been diagnosed for nearly a year, others for a matter of just a few weeks. There was plenty of time for people to get to know each other, to compare experiences, and for those with longer experience to encourage and support those who were very new. During each morning, the team (a dietitian, diabetes nurse, psychologist and doctor) facilitated a discussion on specific aspects of managing type 1 diabetes. These included: carbohydrate counting, managing glucose levels, psychological issues and long-term health (all the things that I will cover in the next few chapters). There then followed time for each person to discuss any issues with one of the team individually. This could lead to a further appointment being made with one of the team, according to the need. Each person was asked to attend four consecutive sessions over a one year period, and then moved on to the next stage of the care pathway, which was largely clinic-based reviews plus more intensive education when required.

At each visit to LWD, a blood sample was taken to measure HbA1c and participants were asked to compete the PAID (Problem Areas in Diabetes) questionnaire, which provides an overview of how they are managing emotionally and psychologically with their diabetes. After a few years, we analysed the data. This analysis showed that at the end of the year, HbA1c levels had reduced significantly. Interestingly the best results were in those that had attended all four sessions. This was perhaps to be expected. Something that was not quite so expected was that although the PAID scores were generally very good, they tended to be higher (indicating more problems) mid-way through the year, then improve again. The precise reasons for this are not clear, but I suspect it is something like this: in the immediate period after diagnosis, there is understandable concern about the impact of diabetes, having to manage injections, and the implication for the future, plus the impact of feeling unwell because of high blood glucose. As people learn to manage their diabetes, get back to work and feel better, things improve, but then a little while afterwards the reality of the diagnosis and its possible impact sinks in, perhaps at around six months after diagnosis. It may be that a few hypos have occurred, or other experiences have shaken people's confidence. Whatever the cause, this is the time when under the traditional system, people were often left to fend for themselves. However, with the LWD programme, they are never more than a few weeks away from a routine review and an opportunity to compare notes with others who are going through (or have already been through) the exact same issues and concerns. And this, I feel, is one of the more powerful aspects of such a group, the ability to help people address their concerns by speaking with others, and I have no doubt that this helped improve the PAID scores by the end of the first year of living with diabetes.

Another unexpected bonus of the LWD programme was that as people were taught about how to adjust their insulin doses according to their carbohydrate intake and their blood glucose levels, they started to make their own adjustments independently. This is particularly important for people who enter a honeymoon period, when the pancreas 'wakes up' again for a while and produces some insulin.

This means that the dose injected must be reduced, often quite significantly, otherwise there is a risk of hypoglycaemia. We witnessed many people who, with the skills they had learnt from the programme, did indeed reduce their insulin, and in some cases stopped taking rapid-acting insulin altogether as their own pancreas was producing enough to keep glucose levels controlled during the daytime. This will be covered in more detail in chapter 9.

So, it is not uncommon that people start off needing quite high doses of insulin, to bring their high blood glucose levels down, and then just a few months later need very little insulin indeed, as their pancreas has (temporarily) woken up again. Without the knowledge and skills about how to make these adjustments, I have seen some people stay on the initial high doses and then find they had to eat extra to 'mop up' the excess insulin and keep their glucose levels from falling too low. This risked causing weight gain and, in some cases, unfortunately led to a really bad hypo.

A few years ago, Dr Sarita Naik was part of our team in Bournemouth and she conducted some interviews with people who had been through the LWD programme, and also with some who had attended a more traditional clinic service at another hospital. These identified five key areas where the LWD programme appeared to have helped those that attended it: Adjustment, Freedom, Control, Support and Knowledge.[15] I think it is worth exploring each of these in a little detail.

Adjustment

As with many individuals with diabetes, the participants completing LWD commented on the difficult time they had at diagnosis and the distress at receiving the diagnosis. The early months after diagnosis were daunting. However, they all felt that a year later they were coping well and coming to terms with the diagnosis. Some of the individuals felt that they had learnt to make the necessary changes to their lifestyle so that they could live as normal a life as possible alongside their diabetes.

In contrast, those who received conventional treatment were more likely to comment on the difficulties they were facing and the day-to-day problems that occurred. For one person this resulted in feelings of depression. They said they were *just existing but no life. It is just existing for the sheer hell of it. That's what it means to me.*

Freedom

Carbohydrate counting allows patients to have dietary freedom and maintain near-normal blood glucose levels. All patients who had attended the LWD programme felt that they could eat what they wanted and there were no restrictions to their diet and consequently there were no restrictions to their life. This contributed to the ease with which they were able to cope with their diabetes.

Patients who received conventional treatment had been taught some of the principles of carbohydrate counting although they had not formally attended an education programme. These individuals did not comment on the freedom or flexibility that can be associated with this.

Control

Those who had attended LWD were not afraid to make changes to their diabetes treatment and were able to adjust their insulin appropriately to the situation. They could explore the causes for hypo- or hyperglycaemic episodes and react to them with the most appropriate treatment. As a result, they felt in control of their diabetes and had no fear of hypoglycaemia. All participants had concerns about long-term complications. However, they also felt that they had the ability to control their diabetes and reduce the risks of complications in the future. The individuals involved in the study were targeting good control and felt this was not only achievable but was also possible to maintain. One said, '*When I am swimming I have got the confidence to change things. I know what to do when I am high. I know I come down by doing extra insulin, how to calculate carbohydrates. I don't have a problem.*'

On the other hand, those that attended the conventional clinic were more likely to describe periods of poor control. This often resulted in feelings of frustration and worries about long-term complications. One person described the frustration at their inability to manage when they developed a cold: '*I had a bad cold and I changed jobs all within two weeks and suddenly my diabetes went out of control ... no matter what I seemed to do I just couldn't get it back in control and I got very frustrated with it. I almost got quite low over it then. Suddenly I had this thing that no matter what I do, I cannot seem to get this right.*'

Support

There are two aspects to this theme. These were peer support and the support from healthcare professionals. Those who attended LWD felt that they were able to learn from other peoples' experiences and solve their problems in the small group discussions. They believed that their experiences were more likely to be acknowledged and validated by others who had diabetes than with healthcare professionals. The programme was also thought to be an 'open forum' and as such allowed the participants' agenda to be followed rather than that of the healthcare professionals. They felt that the LWD sessions allowed all their questions to be answered over the year. As one said, *'It was very helpful because you also come along to these classes and meet people who have had it for longer and you think how well they have coped with it. I have learnt a lot from them. They would say how they felt and I would think, "Oh yes, that's me."'*

While the participants who had conventional treatment felt that they had received good support from their healthcare professionals at diagnosis, they were more likely to describe problems which occurred about six months from diagnosis and it was at this point that they felt that less support was available. One said: *'I felt that over time somebody would teach me a bit more and then I went to my first six-monthly check-up, expecting for people to say "Right, now we will teach you the next bit." And nobody did so when it started going wrong, yes – I did make a few phone calls, yes – people did call me back and say, "We'll try this, we'll try that and see if it works." But nobody has actually educated me on diabetes.'*

Knowledge

All participants who attended LWD thought that they had developed a good knowledge and understanding of the key diabetes issues over the year. They felt that it can be difficult to take in some of the facts shortly after diagnosis. However, the sessions took place over the year and that allowed participants to accumulate that knowledge at their own pace. One person commented: *'I have not come across anything which I think, "I wonder why nobody told me about that," because we have had three-monthly meetings – you have got every opportunity to get all the information that you think you might want.'*

To summarise, by providing **Support** and **Knowledge**, LWD enabled people with newly diagnosed type 1 diabetes to **Adjust** to their new diagnosis, **Control** their diabetes and as a result experience **Freedom** in their lifestyles.

That is my hope for you as you read this book, especially if you have been diagnosed with type 1 diabetes in the last few months. While some centres have set up a similar programme to LWD, many have not and so I hope that by reading this book, and learning how and when to make use of the expertise from your diabetes team, you too will gain the **Support** and **Knowledge** you need to **Adjust** to your diabetes, get it under **Control** and as a result experience **Freedom** in your lifestyle.

6

LEARNING ABOUT CARBOHYDRATES

Following the diagnosis of type 1 diabetes, the important first steps are to get established on insulin treatment and regular blood glucose monitoring, as we discussed in the last chapter. The next task is to begin to learn how different foods affect blood glucose levels. The reason for this is not then to produce a list of 'banned foods' but so that you can understand the impact of what you eat on your blood glucose level, and so that you know how much insulin to take to offset that impact. You may then decide to restrict those foods which have the biggest impact on your glucose levels.

While a number of different food types can affect your blood glucose level, the foods that have the most direct impact are sugars and starches, which are both types of carbohydrate. The most basic type of carbohydrate is a sugar called glucose. Another that you will probably have heard of is fructose, a very similar molecule found in fruit. Some sugars are made up of a combination of two types of sugar molecule. Sucrose (or table sugar) is glucose and fructose; lactose (milk sugar) is glucose and galactose, and maltose (often found in manufactured bread and cereal products) is two glucose molecules joined together. Starches are simply lots of glucose molecules strung together. Once in the body they quickly fall apart into separate glucose molecules. Therefore, it is really important that you have a good understanding of which foods contain sugar and starch, as generally these are the foods for which you will need to take insulin.

You may have been advised that it is important to base all meals on starchy carbohydrates. As mentioned earlier, this is because the official UK nutrition advice for the general population is to do just that.[16] You might think that someone with diabetes should receive different advice (as all starches are essentially glucose) but in their wisdom, the powers that be decided in the 1990s that people with diabetes should receive the same nutritional advice as the general population. And, in the UK, official Government nutritional advice for everyone, not just those with diabetes (as the extract taken from the 'NHS Choices: Eight tips for healthy eating' web page makes clear), is that everyone should include starchy carbohydrates in every meal:

'Base your meals on starchy carbohydrates. Starchy carbohydrates should make up just over one third of the food you eat. They include potatoes, bread, rice, pasta and cereals. Choose wholegrain varieties (or eat potatoes with their skins on) when you can: they contain more fibre, and can make you feel full for longer. Most of us should eat more starchy foods: try to include at least one starchy food with each main meal. Some people think starchy foods are fattening, but gram for gram they contain fewer than half the calories of fat.'

Note the last sentence that a gram of carbohydrate contains fewer than half the calories of a gram of fat. That is certainly true, but does I think miss the crucial point that encouraging a carbohydrate-based diet can mean that the amount of carbohydrate eaten can easily be over twice that of fat, thus cancelling out the benefit of carbohydrates containing fewer calories. In recent years, more and more people have questioned the wisdom of this approach for the general population. In people without diabetes, a high intake of starch leads to the pancreas secreting high levels of insulin – and it is high insulin levels that are known to be fattening. Increasingly therefore, many people in the diabetes community are becoming convinced that this advice is positively wrong for them. And it is easy to understand why. All starchy carbohydrate is broken down in the gut into glucose, which is absorbed into the bloodstream where, in someone with diabetes, it will cause the glucose level to rise. So, every slice of bread, every portion of chips, every portion of rice will cause blood glucose levels to rise – before we even consider the effect of sugars in desserts, cakes, biscuits or cookies. And in someone with type 1 diabetes, all these foods will require insulin, sometimes in high doses, to keep glucose levels down. Those high insulin levels, in turn, risk causing unnecessary weight gain and increased risk of hypoglycaemia. Thus, the traditional dietary advice for people with diabetes makes it difficult to achieve its main goal – normal levels of glucose in the blood.

So, while learning about which foods in your diet contain carbohydrate, I would encourage you to consider how you can cut down on the amount of starch as well as sugar in your diet. That will not only help keep your blood glucose more stable, it will enable you to do so with lower insulin doses, which is also good for your future health.

For now, the focus should be on ensuring that you know how much carbohydrate you are eating, so that you can work out the appropriate dose of insulin to take with your meals. (In chapter 12, we will look in more detail about the benefits of different dietary approaches to managing type 1 diabetes.)

FOODS CONTAINING SUGAR

In order to know how much carbohydrate there is in the food you are eating, the first task is to know which foods contain carbohydrate. As I mentioned, carbohydrates (or carbs for short) are usually divided into sugars and starches. Many people think it is quite obvious which foods have sugar in them, and can reel off a list that looks something like this: sweets, biscuits, cookies, cakes, jam, desserts, ice cream and soda or fizzy drinks. Less obvious perhaps are breakfast cereals (even so-called healthy ones can have a lot of sugar in them) and fruit juice, which is often marketed as natural and healthy. In fact it is not, and should be avoided just like any other sugar-sweetened beverage. Then there are less obvious foods, such as ready meals, take-aways, smoothies, baked beans and just about any processed food you can think of. Even many pizzas are coated with high fructose corn syrup (HFCS) to give them an attractive golden glaze – it is another type of sugar, and potentially quite a harmful one. HFCS (it is also known under many different names on food labels) is a derivative from the production of corn that is commonly found in food and drinks in the US. It is similar to sucrose (a common table sugar that is 50 per cent glucose and 50 per cent fructose), but has at least 10 per cent more fructose than sucrose. In the US, it is much cheaper to produce HFCS than normal sugar and consequently is used in many manufactured foods and drinks. It is used less in the UK and some other European countries. However, in countries with a high HFCS usage, the population is exposed to an extra 10–30 per cent fructose. A recent study has shown that in those countries there are about 20 per cent more cases of (type 2) diabetes than in those who do not use

HFCS.[17] One possible explanation is that fructose is taken up into the liver and it has been shown that excess fructose leads to more internal body fat being laid down – especially in the liver. Excess fat in the liver contributes to the development of type 2 diabetes and the damaging effect of fructose on the liver has been compared to the effect of alcohol.[18] And yet fructose is often cited as being natural, healthy and safe!

Although fructose does not contribute to the development of type 1 diabetes, its effect in possibly causing excess fat to accumulate in the liver is not good for anyone, and to my mind is a good enough reason to minimise it as much as possible. Some 'diabetic' foods contain fructose as it does not directly raise blood glucose – I would suggest you avoid them. Any food that contains HFCS should also be eaten as little as possible. And of course, table sugar (sucrose) is 50 per cent fructose and so, quite apart from its effect on blood glucose levels, it is a good idea to reduce intake of sugar because of the fructose it contains.

The other name for fructose is 'fruit sugar' as it is found in most fruits. However, in fruits, the fructose content is generally small, and the fibre in fruit means it is absorbed much more slowly. Fruit and vegetables are generally considered healthy and often lumped together in health messages. We are all aware of the recommendation to eat a minimum of five portions of fruit and vegetables every day, as explained in the following excerpt from the NHS UK Choices website on what counts towards your 5-a-day:[19]

▶ *80g of fresh, **canned** and/or frozen fruit and vegetables counts as one 5-A-Day portion. Opt for tinned or canned fruit and vegetables in natural juice or water, with no added sugar or salt.*

▶ *30g of **dried fruit** (this is equivalent to around 80g fresh fruit) counts as one 5-A-Day portion. Dried fruit should be eaten at* *mealtimes, not as a between-meal snack, to reduce the risk of tooth decay.*

♦ *150ml **fruit juice**, vegetable juice or smoothie. Limit the amount you drink to a combined total of 150ml a day. Crushing fruit and vegetables into juice and smoothies releases the sugars contained in the fruit and vegetables, which can cause damage to teeth.*

Now canned fruit, fruit juice and dried fruit are all high in sugar and not ideal for someone who is looking to reduce their sugar content. What becomes clear is that whatever criteria were used to determine what counts towards your 5-a-day, they certainly did not take into account the sugar content.

Even no-added-sugar juice or tinned fruits are not a good idea. My own view is that fruit juice should not be included in the 5-a-day list, unless taken in very small quantities, as most of the bits that make fruit healthy have been removed: a 200ml (8oz) glass of orange juice contains 112 calories, 21g of sugar and only 0.1g of fibre. A whole orange, on the other hand, only contains 45 calories and 9g of sugar while providing 2.3g of dietary fibre. Smoothies, also marketed as being full of goodness, are even worse. A review by the consumer organization *Which?* found that they contain more calories per 100ml (4oz) than a bottle of Coca-Cola. Nearly half the smoothies contained 30g or more of sugar per 250ml (10oz) serving, the equivalent of six teaspoons of sugar.[20]For anyone wishing to achieve stable control of type 1 diabetes, this message needs to be amended to steer people away from sugary foods. I would recommend avoiding fruit juices and smoothies completely and to never drink them to quench your thirst. I would also suggest avoiding dried fruit, except in very small quantities (for example a few raisins in some unsweetened yoghurt) because when the water is removed to produce dried fruit, it leaves it with a very high sugar content. Tropical fruits such as bananas, pineapple and mangoes are also high in sugar and should not be eaten on a regular basis. Suitable 'low sugar' fruits for someone with diabetes are berries (which have a very low sugar content) and a small apple, pear, peach or citrus fruit such as a tangerine, i.e. whole fruit that you can hold in your hand.

Many vegetables on the other hand contain very little sugar and, in the case of leafy vegetables, very little starch, but they do contain plenty of vitamins and minerals and fibre – all good stuff.

FOODS CONTAINING STARCH

While most vegetables contain much less sugar than fruit, they differ greatly in the amount of starch they contain depending on the type. It is therefore best to consider vegetables in four broad categories: 'fruit' vegetables, leafy vegetables, root vegetables and legumes (peas and beans).

Salad vegetables such as tomatoes, cucumber and red and green peppers are in fact the fruits of the plant as they contain the seeds. However, they are generally eaten as vegetables. They all have quite low sugar content and can be eaten freely.

Leafy vegetables are generally from plants where we eat the green leaves that grow above ground. Examples include broccoli, cabbage, spinach, lettuce and cauliflower. These are all rich in fibre and vitamin C, with very low sugar or starch content, and can be eaten in unlimited quantities.

Root vegetables are those where we eat the roots, such as all types of potatoes, carrots, turnips, parsnips and beetroots. These roots store energy for the plant that helps them to survive as they lie dormant over winter. Much of this energy is in the form of starchy carbohydrate and for this reason anyone with diabetes should eat root vegetables in moderation. Some – such as onions, carrots and swedes – are about 10 per cent carbohydrate, so a small portion will contain very little carbohydrate. Potato and parsnips are nearer 20 per cent and should only be eaten in small quantities. Beetroot is 10 per cent carbohydrate of which 7 per cent is sugar.

Legumes are a class of vegetable that produce beans that are either eaten alone (such as peas or broad beans) or together with their 'pods' such as French beans, runner beans or sugar snap peas. Their carbohydrate content varies considerably and so it is important to know which ones are high and which are low in carbohydrate.

Any that are eaten with their pods are low in carbohydrate and can be eaten freely. Split peas and chickpeas contain about 40 per cent and 50 per cent carbohydrate respectively, and are best avoided as they are often eaten in quite large quantities. Lentils, black-eye beans and kidney beans are better options, but still contain around 20 per cent carbohydrate.

Garden peas are relatively low in carbohydrate, however beware mushy peas that are very dense and can contain much more carbohydrate that you might think. Sweetcorn is strictly speaking a grain, but is often viewed as a vegetable similar to peas. However, it contains around 20 per cent carbohydrate and anything more than a small portion will increase your glucose level.

Grains are foods that come from wheat, rice, oats, barley or other cereal grains. They are rich in carbohydrates, and all types of bread, pasta, rice and breakfast cereals fall into this category. Grains are classified either as whole grains or refined grains. Whole grains are recommended as they contain dietary fibre, iron and a number of B vitamins. Examples include wholemeal flour, brown rice and wholemeal pasta. Refined grains have been milled, a process that removes the fibre, iron and vitamins, to produce white flour, white rice or pasta. When the fibre is removed by way of the refining process, it increases the glycaemic index, meaning these products will have a greater effect on blood glucose levels.

For people with diabetes, wholegrains are to be preferred. While many people enjoy wholemeal bread, many find wholemeal pasta, for example, unappetizing; and some people with irritable bowel syndrome may not be able to eat wholegrains that contain insoluble fibre. It is also important to remember that a large portion of bread, rice or pasta will have a big effect on your glucose levels, regardless of the type – it is just that the wholemeal variety will lead to a more prolonged effect than white bread. The advice therefore, is to aim to reduce your intake of bread, rice or pasta. This is best done by avoiding meals that are based on these foods, such as sandwiches, pasta or rice dishes, and when you do eat them, have them as a small component of the meal, rather than the basis for the whole meal.

All breakfast cereals are made from grains and therefore are high in carbohydrate – even 'healthy' ones such as porridge oats or bran flakes. So quite apart from their sugar content, the starch in breakfast cereals will mean that they will increase your blood glucose level and require a hefty insulin dose.

To summarise: in order to help control your diabetes it is important to know which foods contain carbohydrates and to reduce them where possible. That means reducing (and avoiding where possible) all sweet foods, together with breakfast cereals, bread, rice and pasta plus some fruits and vegetables. In this regard, it is important not to lump all fruit and vegetables together, as current recommendations do. Focus on eating those that will have the least effect on your glucose levels, such as:

- Berries
- Leafy and salad vegetables
- Mange tout and French or runner beans.

The following can be eaten in moderation:

- Apples, pears, citrus fruit, peaches
- Carrots and swedes
- Peas, lentils and kidney beans.

And these should be eaten in small quantities only:

- Banana, pineapple, melon
- Potatoes, parsnips and chick peas
- Bread, rice, pasta and breakfast cereals.

Fruit juice and smoothies should be avoided altogether. However, if you really enjoy these have a small glass and enjoy the texture and flavour. Don't drink them to quench your thirst or to satisfy hunger.

PRACTICAL STEPS TO REDUCE CARBOHYDRATE IN YOUR DIET

First, I would like you to engage in my ten-minute consultation on reducing carbohydrates. It goes something like this. Ask yourself:

- What do you generally eat for breakfast?
- For lunch?
- For your evening meal?
- For snacks?

Typical answers will include cereal and toast for breakfast, perhaps with orange juice, a sandwich or baguette for lunch, maybe with a packet of crisps, and an apple or banana for a snack, or maybe digestive biscuits. Followed by a variety of meals in the evening that usually includes potatoes, rice or pasta, which are all carbohydrates of course.

My first suggestion is to avoid cereals at breakfast and to try a breakfast based on eggs (cooked any way, with bacon, tomatoes, mushrooms and with or without one thin slice of toast) or natural yoghurt. I find Greek yoghurt nicer (it has a high protein content and is up to 10 per cent fat!) mixed with a handful of berries, nuts or seeds and perhaps some oats. And, please, no fruit juice.

Lunch could be a home-made soup (avoiding starchy vegetables like potatoes and parsnips) or a salad, and while evening meals can include some starch, such as bread, rice, potato or pasta, it should occupy just a small corner of the plate if at all, while most of the plate is filled with green vegetables or salad. Or try a meal with just meat and green vegetables. So, as a rule, it is best to avoid meals based on carbohydrates such as potato or pasta bake, macaroni cheese, pizza or rice dishes. But if you really enjoy these dishes, have them as an occasional treat and know you will need an appropriately large insulin dose for them.

For snacks, an apple, tangerine, peach, plum or pear are fine (i.e. any small 'round' fruit you can fit in the palm of your hand. Berries are very low in sugar. It is best to avoid eating bananas (unless a small one), pineapple or melon on a regular basis. Try to make up your five-a-day from vegetables rather than fruit. But you could also try a hard-boiled egg, a small piece of cheese or a handful of nuts, which apart from peanuts and cashews contain hardly any carbohydrates, but plenty of healthy fats.

With only this modest information to hand, many people have achieved much better control of their diabetes. What is interesting is that by following this advice, people often find they are eating more fresh and natural foods, and less processed food. This means they are also eating less sugar and salt as they are to be found in worrying quantities in just about every type of processed food.

PORTION SIZE

It is well established that over the years, portion sizes have increased. This not only applies to pre-prepared food but also, as food has become more available and affordable, to home-served foods. The old 'regular' serving of French fries in fast-food restaurants is now 'small'; confectionary bars have got larger (although in recent years there has been some reversal of this trend) and muffins and cookies are now often big enough to share. By now, it will be obvious that we don't actually need all this extra food. Whereas in previous generations, the challenge was to get enough to eat, now the challenge is to limit what we eat. There are certain foods, such as green vegetables, that do not need to be limited, but in the context of controlling blood glucose levels, limiting carbohydrates is essential. As a general rule, I would suggest aiming for no more than about 25–30g of carbohydrate with each meal. Now this doesn't mean that you have to eat carbohydrate with every meal, and it is possible to survive very well (and improve blood glucose control) by having a very low, or no-carbohydrate meal for one or two meals a day. On the other hand, you may occasionally have a larger portion of carbohydrates as a special treat, for example. However, this will likely cause a rise in blood glucose levels over the next few hours, even with extra insulin.

The table below gives examples of different portion sizes of carbohydrates for different meals. This is not an exhaustive list, but is aimed at giving you an idea of how much a certain amount of carbohydrate looks like. I am very grateful to Chris Cheyette for providing this information, and would recommend his *Carbs & Cals* book (or its smartphone app) as a very useful resource to help you learn more about carbohydrate portion size.[21]

Examples of meals of different carbohydrate content

Carbo-hydrate	Breakfast	Lunch	Dinner	Snack
10g or less	1. Whole grapefruit with or without sweetener 2. Natural yoghurt (60g) with straw-berries (80g) 3. 2-egg omelette with mushrooms	1. Mackerel salad with beetroot and horseradish 2. Vegetable soup (no potatoes) 3. Chicken salad	1. Tuna steak with steamed vegetables 2. Vegetable and bean stew 3. Prawn stir fry with pineapple pieces	1. Apple 2. Plain Popcorn (20g) 3. Almonds (30g)
20g	1. 4 small breakfast **pancakes** with cherry tomatoes 2. Scrambled egg on 1 slice thick **toast** 3. **Branflakes** (20g) with **milk**	1. Small slice **quiche** (100g) with salad 2. Smoked salmon on ½ **bagel** 3. 3 **Ryvita** with low-fat cream cheese	1 **Shepherds pie (200g) with vegetables** 2. Chilli con **carne with nachos (20g)** 3. Steak with grilled mushrooms and **new potatoes (100g)**	1. Medium **banana** 2. **Houmous and** vegetable sticks 3. **Cereal bar**
30g	1. **All Bran (40g) with milk** 2. 2 slices medium **toast** with peanut butter 3. **Eggs benedict**	1. 1 tin **tomato soup** 2. Medium **wholegrain roll** with sliced turkey and salad 3. 3 bean **wrap**	4. **Lasagne (225g) with** salad 5. Chicken stir fry with **egg noodles (80g)** 6. Baked salmon with small **jacket potato** and vegetables	1 **Coffee & walnut cake (50g)** 2. **Hot cross bun** 3. 2 scoops ice cream

Carbo-hydrate	Breakfast	Lunch	Dinner	Snack
40g	1. Breakfast pancakes 2. 2 Oatabix with milk 3. No added sugar muesli (50g) with milk	1. Ham salad sandwich 2. Cous cous salad 3. 1 tin mushroom soup with 2 medium slices bread	1. Mushroom risotto (240g) 2. Chicken and broccoli pasta (340g) 3. Beef stew with 2 small dumplings	1. Malt loaf (60g) 2. Mince pie (60g) 3. Dates (60g)
50g	1. 2 slices thick toast with jam 2. Large bowl porridge made with milk (350g) 3. Croissant with marmalade and glass orange juice	1. Baked beans on toast 2. 6 pieces of sushi 3. Pasta salad	1. 2 slices deep pan pizza 2. Lentil curry with brown rice (95g) 3. Tuna pasta bake (350g)	1. Flapjack (80g) 2. Large hot chocolate drink 3. Medium Easter egg (100g)

Each cell gives three examples of meals for each type and carbohydrate content. The carbohydrate-containing part of the meal is shown in **bold**. Note how even 'healthy' cereals can push breakfast to 30g of carbohydrate or more and how some snacks (e.g. a flapjack) can contain 50g of carbohydrate, whereas some main meals (such as shepherd's pie) might only contain 20g.

GLYCAEMIC INDEX

We have established that avoiding high carbohydrate meals will help. This does not mean you should necessarily avoid carbohydrate altogether, although some do advocate a very low carbohydrate diet, as we will discuss in chapter 12. What is important is that wherever possible the carbohydrate eaten should have as little effect on blood glucose levels as possible.

This is where the concept of glycaemic index (GI) comes in. Some foods are absorbed very quickly which, in turn, causes the glucose level in the blood to rise sharply – these food types are termed 'high GI' foods; other types of food that are absorbed more slowly are termed 'low GI' foods. The glycaemic index of glucose itself is 100. The GI of orange juice is 50, which means that its effect on the blood glucose level is equivalent to half the effect of eating glucose. The table below shows the GI for a number of common foods. It can be seen, for example, that a baguette has a very high GI of 95, whereas rye bread has a GI of just 58. Similarly, boiled potatoes have a GI of 50, whereas a baked potato has a GI of 85. Using this information will help you learn how to still enjoy eating bread or potatoes – by choosing types that have a low GI.

The overall effect of a food on your blood glucose level will not depend merely on its glycaemic index, but also on how much of it you eat. For example, a very small piece of baguette (high GI) will have a much smaller effect on blood glucose level than a whole plateful of boiled potatoes, even though they have a lower GI. Thus, at the end of the day it is the total amount of carbohydrate that will affect your blood glucose levels. Therefore, the key message is to stick to small portions of low GI foods wherever possible and to avoid high GI foods as much as you can.

Glycaemic Index of common foods

BREAD	
Baguette	95
White bread – wheat	70
Rye bread – wholemeal	58

PASTA/RICE	
Basmati rice	58
White rice	64
Brown rice	55
Pasta – durum wheat	44
Pasta – wholewheat	37
SWEET FOODS	
Scone	92
Doughnut	76
Ice cream	61
Mars bar	65
Digestive biscuit	59
BEVERAGES	
Coca cola	53
Orange juice	50
Tomato juice	38
BREAKFAST CEREALS	
Cornflakes	81
All Muesli	40–66
Bran	42
FRUIT	
Figs (dried)	61
Sultanas	60
Banana	52
Grapes	46
Peach	42
Strawberries	40
Apple	38

Pear	38
LEGUMES	
Baked beans	48
Butter beans	31
Green lentils	30
Chick peas	28
Kidney beans	28
VEGETABLES	
Parsnips	97
Baked potato	85
Chips	75
Mashed potato	74
Beetroot	64
Carrots – cooked	58
Boiled potato	50
Peas	48
Carrots – raw	16

NAUGHTY BUT NICE

This section covers sweet foods such as cakes, biscuits/cookies, pastries, sweets/candy, chocolate, ice cream and desserts. They all contain sugar and will influence your glucose levels. Apart from sugar, they also contain fat and anything other than a small portion will have a high calorie content.

These foods do not serve any nutritional purpose and, simply put, we do not need to eat them. In an ideal world, they are best avoided completely, and if you do not have a sweet tooth this may well be the best and easiest option. However, they are often very tasty, and regularly feature as part of many social events, such as birthday celebrations, a meal out or even that ice cream on a hot sunny day. So, if you do have a sweet tooth, make the effort to learn the carbohydrate content of your favourite sweet foods and find out how much you can get away with without it having a big effect on your glucose levels. The *Carbs & Cals* book is again very useful for this purpose. This will tell you, for example, that you can enjoy a small ice cream or portion of banoffee pie and only consume around 20g of carbohydrates. However, if you are anything like me, restricting yourself to a small portion will require a huge amount of willpower. It is best not to have these foods in your house, but enjoy them now and again as a treat when you are eating out.

One tip for chocolate lovers: have some really good quality dark chocolate in the house; break it up into squares and keep it in a container. Not only does dark chocolate contain all sorts of chemicals that are good for you, but unless you are a complete chocoholic, it is very difficult to eat a large quantity of it. It also has much lower sugar content than milk chocolate and is consequently a lot less moreish.

CARBOHYDRATE COUNTING

By now, you will have some idea of what foods contain carbohydrate. The next step is to learn how to estimate how much carbohydrate there is in the foods that you eat. To do this precisely is quite difficult, but at this stage, it is sufficient to start with a few basic tips to get you started. The table below provides a 'beginners' guide. Note it includes some of the foods that I have advised you to avoid as part of your routine, just in case you do choose to eat them now and again.

For much greater detail, the *Carbs & Cals* book and app provides a very easy-to-use guide to counting carbs and covers a huge range of different foods. If you don't already have it, I would recommend you download the app so you have it all in your phone and with you all the time.

Food Portion	Carbohydrate (g)
Medium slice of bread	15
Medium bread roll	25
1in/2.5cm French stick	10
1 pitta bread	30
1 Weetabix	10
30g (5tbsp) Corn flakes	25
30g (7tbsp) Rice Krispies	25
30g (4tbsp) Branflakes/Fruit 'n Fibre	20
30g (2tbsp) Muesli (no added sugar)	20
35g (1tbsp) cooked rice	10
50g (½cup) cooked pasta	10
1 egg size portion (60g) boiled potato	10
30g (5 medium) chips	10
120g (3tbsp) baked beans	15
½ thin crust pizza	50
Medium apple/pear/orange	15
Medium banana	20
200ml (7fl oz) pure fruit juice	20
200ml (7fl oz) milk	10
125g ($^1/_4$cup) low fat yoghurt	15
125g ($^1/_4$cup) plain Greek yoghurt	6
1 Digestive biscuit	10
2 Rich Tea biscuits	10
2 Jaffa Cakes	15
1 doughnut	25
65g (standard size) Mars Bar	45
25g (1 small) packet crisps	15
3 Dextrosol Tablets	10
100ml (4fl oz) Lucozade	10

When you start out with carbohydrate counting, reading food labels on packaged food can be very important. However, it is important to know exactly what you are looking for. In the UK and the US, food labels differ but they both show the grams of carbohydrate and of sugar per serving size. It is also important that you use the number given for total carbohydrates (that includes all sugars and starches) rather than just the figure for sugars, as of course the starch also is converted into glucose.

Also remember to compare the serving size stated on the label to the amount you would eat. If it is a small pack of crisps/chips or a sandwich and there is one serving in the pack, and you eat it all, then it is quite straightforward. The carbohydrate you eat is the amount per serving. It becomes more complicated when you have a tub of ice cream, that says it contains 10 servings, yet you usually eat half the tub at a time. In that case you will have eaten five standard servings, and so you will have to multiply the carbohydrates per serving by 5 to calculate your total carbohydrate intake.

As your glucose levels come under control after you have been diagnosed, you will need to start adjusting your mealtime insulin dose according to the carbohydrates you are eating. As a rule, I suggest you use one unit of mealtime insulin for every 10 grams of carbohydrate in the meal you are about to eat. However, if your total insulin dose for the day (including basal insulin) is less than 30 units, then start with 0.5 units for every 10 grams of carbohydrate. This should ensure that you do not accidentally give yourself too much insulin, and as you begin to reduce your carbohydrate intake, you will automatically reduce your insulin dose.

The BERTIE online e-learning programme is a great resource to learn about carbohydrate counting. Note that neither this, nor the *Carbs & Cals* book, specifically encourage a low-carbohydrate diet, but the principles involved are very useful in learning how to count your carbohydrates. And they do a much better job than I can in a book such as this.

7

MEASURING BLOOD GLUCOSE LEVELS

SELF-BLOOD GLUCOSE MONITORING (SBGM)

The aim in managing type 1 diabetes is to achieve blood glucose values that are as near to normal as possible. In someone with normal glucose metabolism this will generally mean a value of no more than 5.5mmol/l (100mg/dl) while fasting (such as first thing in the morning) and before meals, and no more than 7.8mmol/l (140mg/dl) after meals. This chapter will address how you can monitor your progress in achieving good control of diabetes and make sure you are on track to achieve your goals.

Until the late 1980s, the only method available for a person with diabetes to monitor their diabetic control was by checking the level of glucose in their urine. This involved peeing into a container and dipping a plastic strip with chemicals embedded at one end into the urine. The chemicals reacted with the glucose in the urine, causing the colour of the strip to change according to the amount of glucose in the urine. The colour was then compared with a colour chart to give an indication of how much glucose was present. Such strips are still available and similar strips are also available to check the level of protein and ketones and many other constituents in the urine.

Before the development of strips in the 1970s, checking the glucose in the urine involved peeing into a container, then adding tablets containing the chemicals and observing the colour change and before this the technique involved boiling the urine! Urine test strips are therefore a huge advance on what was previously available. They are cheap and easy to use, but unfortunately not appropriate for intensive management of diabetes, for the following reasons:

1. Urine testing relies on the kidneys excreting glucose from the urine when levels in the blood rise too high. However, glucose generally does not appear in the urine until the level in the blood is over 10mmol/l or 180mg/dl, which is much too high for anyone aiming for good control of his or her diabetes. In some people, especially in the elderly, glucose levels can rise even higher before appearing in the urine.

2. Urine is constantly formed by the kidneys and then passes into the bladder where it is stored until a person next urinates, which could be several hours later. Consequently, a urine test is always 'out of date' and does not reflect the level of glucose in the blood at the time the urine is tested.

3. Urine testing, by definition, means that you have to have some urine in your bladder to pee, and that you can find a loo.

As urine test strips were developed, similar technology was used to develop strips that measured the level of glucose in the blood. The earliest strips changed colour according to the blood glucose level, and were read in the same way as urine test strips. By the late 1980s meters became available that read the colour change automatically and gave a digital read-out of the result. However, the testing routine was still quite cumbersome: one of the most popular tests required the person to prick their finger and squeeze a drop of blood onto the end of the strip; they then had to wait exactly 60 seconds before wiping the blood off the strip, and then wait another 60 seconds to read the colour of the strip by comparing it with a colour chart printed on the side of the container for the strips. Subsequently, meters were developed that read strips automatically. Nowadays many meters produce an accurate result in about five seconds.

Blood testing has the obvious disadvantage that you need to prick your finger to get some blood out. If you do lots of tests this can make your fingers quite sore. It can also be quite inconvenient, especially, for example, for people who work in dirty environments, who handle food or who are not easily able to wash their hands (which is a requirement for an accurate result).

Despite these drawbacks blood testing provides an accurate record of the blood glucose level at the precise time the test is done. In fact, checking your blood glucose level is an essential component of taking control of your diabetes, second only to taking insulin. Newer technologies, that remove the need for frequent finger-pricks, are becoming more available and affordable all the time (see chapter 14) but for the foreseeable future, regular finger prick tests are still required.

There are several types of blood glucose meter. In the UK, they are generally available free of charge via diabetes clinics; test strips are also available free on prescription and there should be no limit on the number prescribed (within reason, of course). I do not recommend a particular brand of meter; there is a large range to cater for different needs: some are small and compact, others have larger and easy-to-read displays and some contain the test strips within them. There are also some meters that have a built-in bolus advisor that will do the calculation of your insulin dose for you. These can be very useful for people who are willing to enter the relevant details (such as the carbohydrate content of each meal) each time they test.

WHEN SHOULD YOU TEST YOUR BLOOD GLUCOSE?

As a rule, it is important to test your blood glucose at the following times:

1. <u>When you are about to inject insulin.</u> This is number one for a reason – it is the most important time that you really do need to know your glucose level. It is potentially dangerous to inject insulin if you do not know your current level of blood glucose. Furthermore, intensive management of type 1 diabetes requires that you adjust the dose of insulin if your glucose level is too low or too high (this is covered in more detail in chapter 11). This means that, as a minimum, you should check your blood glucose before each meal (unless it contains no carbohydrate), and before injecting your basal insulin (usually in the evening and/or morning). I sometimes use the acronym 'TIE', which stands for Test – Inject – Eat to encourage people to TIE these three things together and in that order.

2. <u>Before going to bed and first thing in the morning.</u> Often these are times when you would be injecting insulin, but if not, it is still a good idea to check your glucose at these times. Firstly, you can use these tests to check that you are on the right dose of basal insulin. Testing at these times will also enable you to give a correction

dose if the level is too high, or to take some carbohydrate if it is too low. This is especially important at bedtime, when it is important to ensure that you are not hypoglycaemic before going to bed.

3. <u>Before driving or operating machinery.</u> It is essential that you know what your blood glucose level is before driving a car or operating machinery. The main concern here is hypoglycaemia, as a low blood glucose level can severely impair coordination and reaction times, increasing the risk of an accident that might cause injury (or worse) to you or another person. It is acceptable to have tested your blood glucose within two hours before driving, for example if you had a meal an hour before setting off. It is also recommended to test every two hours while on a long journey.

4. <u>Before during and after exercise.</u> Any physical activity (such as walking, shopping, housework) will affect your blood glucose level, and sometimes more than you might anticipate. Again, it makes sense to have checked the level before any period of increased physical activity. It is essential to check blood glucose before and during more active activities such as sports, and this will be covered in more detail in chapter 16.

5. <u>When you are feeling unwell.</u> Any infection or other illness can cause a rise in blood glucose level that might require you to take additional insulin, even if you are off your food. This is even more important if you also have evidence of increased ketones, as explained under 'sick day rules', later in this chapter on page 92. So, if you are feeling unwell, it is important to check your glucose level, and if it is higher than expected, to recheck at least every two hours.

6. <u>After meals</u>. As a rule, it is generally sufficient to check your glucose level before meals, but sometimes it will also be important to do so about two hours afterwards. This will be the

case if you are not entirely sure of the carbohydrate content of what you have eaten (at a restaurant for example) or if you wish to make sure that you are taking the correct dose for your meals. Ideally the level two hours after a meal should be about the same as the level before a meal, or rise by at most 2–3mmol/l (30–50mg/dl).

Having read this, you may be forgiven for thinking that you will be asked to check your glucose levels almost constantly. In practice, for most people, testing between 4 and 6 times a day is often enough, unless you are driving for a long period, feeling unwell or undertaking exercise.

STARTING OFF WITH BLOOD TESTING

It is a good idea to get into the habit of regular testing as soon as you are diagnosed, and to write the results in a record book. As a minimum, it is suggested that you test first thing in the morning, before every insulin injection and before bed. While most meters store your readings, it is much easier for you (and your doctor or nurse) to identify patterns in your results if you write them down in a book. A number of meter and insulin companies produce these, or you can use a small notebook, in which you can divide the pages into columns as below:

Date	Before breakfast	Before lunch	Before dinner	Before bed	Other	Notes

Many meters also have software available that you can use to download and display your results. This can be very helpful to identify patterns and assess whether your insulin doses need adjusting, as will be discussed in chapter 14.

It is important that you do blood tests for your own benefit; that means there must be a good reason for doing them, and that you understand what to do with the results. All too often in the past, people were told to do blood tests, often several times a day, without being given sufficient guidance as to what to do with the results. I well remember many years ago, seeing people in clinic who had dutifully performed many tests – day in, day out – where there were many consistently high or low values, that the person had no ability to act upon. It was as if the main reason was to produce lots of numbers to bring to the next clinic visit.

Thankfully those days are largely behind us, although I still find that some people can get into the habit of doing a test, and then not actually acting upon the result. So, the next section is designed to provide you with the information you need to act upon each and every test result. We will start with the most important immediate goal of blood glucose testing – to ensure you are not hypo.

HYPOGLYCAEMIA - MAKE FOUR THE FLOOR

Hypoglycaemia just means 'low blood glucose' and is defined as any blood glucose level below 4mmol/l or 70mg/dl. As discussed in chapter 3, the phrase 'make four the floor' was coined to remind individuals to keep their glucose levels above 4mmol/l (70mg/dl) at all times. This is to minimise the risk of levels falling too low and especially to avoid the risk of dangerous hypoglycaemia. If any test you perform produces a result that is less than 4, then you need to take note. If it is above 3.5mmol/l (60mg/dl) and you are about to eat, then you probably do not need to do anything different. However, in any other situation, a level below 4mmol/l

(70mg/dl) needs to be corrected to avoid the level falling still further.

Management of hypoglycaemia

In order to increase the low blood glucose levels as soon as possible, the ideal option is a glucose-rich food or drink.

It is recommended that you take 15g fast-acting carbohydrate and then wait 10–15 minutes, re-test and if the glucose level is still below 4mmol/l (70mg/dl), treat again with a further 15g carbohydrate. The table below shows some examples of treatment for hypos:

Treatment	15g Carbohydrate is found in:
Glucose/dextrose tablets	4
Sports Drinks, e.g. Lucozade Sport	225ml (8oz)
Cola-type fizzy drink	150ml (5oz)
Jelly babies	4
Jelly beans	10
Marshmallow	3 (large)
Fruit pastilles	6
Hypo treatment gel, e.g. Glucogel	1.5 tube

Following this immediate treatment, if you are about to eat, then you should take your normal (or a slightly reduced) dose of insulin and eat straight away. If the hypo occurred between meals, it is advisable to have a small snack such as a piece of fruit or a sandwich, with no additional insulin.

Once you have treated the hypo, it is important to try and identify what caused it. The easy bit is that, fundamentally, there is only one reason a person has a hypo – there is too much insulin in their system. The key is to work out why that is the case. Common reasons include:

- Taking too much insulin for the carbohydrate in a meal.
- Having too much basal insulin.
- Being more active than usual.

Any experience of a hypo should be used as an opportunity to review your current insulin doses, especially if you experience recurrent hypos at about the same time of day, or in similar situations. By and large, a hypo first thing in the morning, or several hours after eating, is likely to be due to too much basal insulin; a hypo within three hours of eating is more likely related to the mealtime (bolus) insulin.

If you are newly diagnosed and have high glucose levels, it is not uncommon that quite high doses of insulin will be needed at first. That is because enough insulin needs to be taken that will actually reduce glucose levels and not just keep them stable. Furthermore, insulin tends to be less effective when glucose levels are high. Within a few days to a couple of weeks, glucose levels will come down to near normal. This means that your insulin injections will be more effective in reducing your blood glucose and, also, that you will need just enough insulin to keep your levels stable, rather than having to bring them down further. It is therefore essential that in this situation you are provided with appropriate information about how to reduce your insulin dose, and that you have support from a professional who can advise on a day-to-day basis about the correct dose to take. Otherwise, failure to reduce the dose can lead to a severe hypo. And in my experience, it only takes one severe hypo, particularly in the early stages of living with type 1 diabetes, to have a profound impact on a person's confidence in their ability to manage their diabetes. At worst, it could lead to a tendency to keep glucose levels high, because of a profound fear of hypoglycaemia.

Symptoms of hypoglycaemia

In chapter 3, we discussed the symptoms that typically occur as a result of hypoglycaemia. These include symptoms that develop from the effect of hormones such as adrenaline (causing tremor, sweating, hunger) as it tries to counter the effect of insulin and increase the glucose levels. Other symptoms (including drowsiness and confusion) result from the brain being starved of glucose.

It is important to recall that these symptoms can be quite subtle, or absent altogether, thus I will recap some of the earlier discussion in chapter 3 about hypoglycaemia unawareness. This is less likely if you are recently diagnosed with type 1 diabetes, but is more common if you have had diabetes for many years and/or if you experience frequent and recurrent hypoglycaemia. It is as if the body becomes so used to running on low, that it stops bothering about sending out warning signs. Such hypo unawareness is potentially very dangerous, as it means you can feel you are functioning quite normally, when in fact your glucose level is too low to provide adequate fuel for the brain, and there is a high risk of drowsiness or unconsciousness. Fortunately, we now know that these symptoms can return if hypos are avoided. However, for anyone at risk of hypo unawareness, regular monitoring of blood glucose is essential to pick up and treat a hypo at the earliest opportunity.

RESPONDING TO A HIGH GLUCOSE LEVEL

The next most important goal of glucose monitoring is to respond to a high glucose level. This is almost always as a result of too little insulin being on board (we will discuss one situation when this is not the case – the Somogyi effect, in chapter 11). The response to a high glucose level will vary, depending on the time of day that it is high, and whether you have recently eaten. For example:

1. If your glucose level first thing in the morning is high, and is higher than the level at the previous bedtime, this suggests the dose of basal insulin was not enough. If this is a regular pattern, then it suggests a need to increase the dose of basal insulin.

2. A high glucose level within three hours of a meal, especially if it is higher than the level before the meal, suggests that insufficient mealtime insulin was taken. This could have been due to your underestimating the amount of carbohydrate you have eaten. However, if the estimate was accurate, and if this pattern recurs for the same meal (e.g. at lunchtime) over a few days, then the lunchtime insulin dose, or rather the insulin to carbohydrate ratio may need to be increased.

3. A high level at other times, especially late afternoon or early evening could suggest that the basal insulin from the previous day has run out. This may require a change in the timing of your basal dose, or of the type of insulin used.

More detailed advice on making these changes is provided in chapters 10 and 11. Such changes will hopefully avoid high readings in the future, but in the meantime it is useful to be able to correct a high glucose level straight away. This is in contrast to what people were told in the past, that they should not take extra insulin if their glucose level is high. With the fast-acting analogues now available, it is perfectly safe to take extra to correct a high glucose level, as long as the amount taken is not too much. In my experience, many people have a tendency to give too much insulin if their glucose is high, and that can then cause the opposite problem, i.e. a hypo.

The safest way to correct a high glucose level is to add a correction dose to your next mealtime insulin dose, and this will be discussed in greater detail in chapter 11. However, as a guide to get you started I would suggest a very gentle correction dose that can be calculated as follows:

▶ If your blood glucose is between 10 and 13mmol/l (180–240mg/dl): add 1 unit to your mealtime dose
▶ If your blood glucose is between 13.1 and 17mmol/l (241–300mg/dl): add 2 units to your mealtime dose
▶ If your blood glucose is between 17.1 and 20mmol/l (301–360mg/dl): add 3 units to your mealtime dose

If you find these suggested doses are not enough, then you can adjust the correction doses as described in chapter 11.

SICK DAY RULES

Sometimes, blood glucose levels are high, not because the insulin dose is incorrect, but because of illness. This is because of the effect of infections or illness in causing high blood glucose levels. Sometimes, even a minor cold can cause glucose levels to rise quite markedly.

So if you do feel unwell, it is important to keep a close eye on your glucose level. If it rises above 14mmol/l (250mg/dl) then it is advisable to check for ketones in your urine or blood. You should be provided with a means of checking ketone levels. This is best done using a meter and strips to measure ketone levels in the blood. There are some glucose meters that can also be used with test strips that measure blood ketones.

The alternative and more usual method of measuring ketones is using a urine test strip. This has the same disadvantages as urine glucose monitoring – namely that the ketones detected have accumulated since the last time you passed urine and are therefore not an accurate reflection of the current level of ketones in the blood. However, they are inexpensive, easy to use and will provide enough information to tell you whether you need to seek medical advice. The results are usually expressed as 'negative', 'trace', '+', '++', '+++' and '++++'.

Either method of testing should be available to you on prescription. They are also available via the Diabetes.co.uk website, which provides the following advice on how to interpret a blood ketone result:

Blood ketone level	Approx. equivalent urine ketone test	Indicates
Under 0.6mmol/l	Negative or trace	A normal blood ketone value.
0.6 to 1.5mmol/l	+ or ++	That more ketones are being produced than normal, test again later to see if the value has lowered.
1.6 to 3.0mmol/l	+++	A high level of ketones, and could present a risk of ketoacidosis. It is advisable to contact your healthcare team for advice.
Above 3.0mmol/l	++++	A dangerous level of ketones which will require immediate medical care.

Note that a slight rise in ketone production is normal during a fast as the body switches to burning fat for energy. A blood ketone level less than 1.0mmol/l or a urine result of '+' might simply reflect that you have not eaten for some hours. In this situation, your blood glucose level will usually be normal. However, if you are feeling unwell, and your blood glucose is above 14mmol/l (250mg/dl) and your blood ketone level is above 1mmol/l (or urine ketone is '++' or higher), then you are advised to take the following corrective action:

- Immediately take 4–6 units of your short- or rapid-acting insulin.
- Drink plenty of water and sugar-free fluids.
- Re-check blood glucose and ketone level every 1–2 hours.
- Repeat the above dose until ketone level has fallen below 1mmol/l (blood) or is '+' or lower (urine) and the blood glucose level has fallen to below 10mmol/l (180mg/dl).
- Try to identify the cause of high blood glucose level and seek treatment if necessary, e.g. for infection.
- If high glucose and ketone levels persist, contact your diabetes team for further advice.
- If you are vomiting or become drowsy contact your doctor or local Emergency Department for urgent assessment.

If you feel unwell but your ketone level is less than 1mmol/l (or urine level is negative, trace or '+'), then less insulin will be required. In this situation, you are advised to:

- Take 2–4 units extra of short- or rapid-acting insulin.
- Drink plenty of water or sugar-free fluids.
- Re-check your glucose level every 2 hours, and if it is above 14mmol/l (250mg/dl) then repeat a ketone test. If this is above 1mmol/l in blood (or '++' in urine), follow the advice in the box above. If ketones are less than this, take an additional 2–4 units of rapid acting insulin until the blood glucose level has fallen to below 10mmol/l.
- Try to find cause of high blood glucose levels and seek treatment or advice.

Further advice on managing periods of illness is provided on page 210 in chapter 15.

LONG-TERM MONITORING OF YOUR DIABETES – HBA1C

As discussed in chapter 2, glycated haemoglobin (abbreviated as HbA1c), is used to assess glucose levels over a longer period, and for many years has been the gold standard means of assessing diabetic control. Its measurement involves a simple blood test that can be taken at any time of day (as it reflects glucose control over the past 6–8 weeks).

In people without diabetes, glycated haemoglobin is generally below 40mmol/mol (5.8 per cent). In a person with type 1 diabetes, a level of 53mmol/mol (7 per cent) or below is indicative of good control; levels much above 64mmol/mol (8 per cent) significantly increase the risk of developing diabetes-related complications. Conversely, levels much lower than 53mmol/mol (7 per cent) can be associated with increased risk of hypoglycaemia. However, a person who manages their diabetes intensively, with multiple injections or an insulin pump and with frequent monitoring, can safely achieve a near normal HbA1c.

It is recommended that HbA1c is checked at least every three months, in order to guide you and your diabetes team in keeping your diabetes under control. It forms part of the follow up of everyone with diabetes.

PERSEVERING WITH BLOOD TESTING

From the above, you will see how important regular blood testing is to help ensure glucose levels are kept as near normal as possible. However, I have met many people with type 1 diabetes, who despite a great start and the best of intentions, fall out of the habit of regularly checking their blood glucose, or stop doing it altogether. I can fully understand why this might happen. Doing a blood test is generally not painful, but over time it can make your fingertips quite sore. It can be a bit messy, you can get blood on your clothes, and it can take a minute or two for the finger to stop bleeding after each test. People whose results are often high can become discouraged, especially if they do not know how to bring their glucose levels down, and in some cases this can lead to them stopping doing tests altogether. Even without these reasons, persevering with regular blood testing requires discipline and a high level of organisation to ensure that you always have your testing kit with you when you need it.

Some people who are quite happy to give themselves several insulin injections every day find it much more difficult to keep up with blood testing. I for one will admit – and I have done on many occasions to people who struggle with regular blood testing – that I would have difficulty finding the discipline and organisation necessary to do all the blood tests that would be necessary if I had type 1 diabetes.

Earlier in this chapter, I said that blood testing is second only to taking insulin in its importance in the management of type 1 diabetes. Thus, if you ever find yourself in the situation where you are not doing regular tests, or you have stopped altogether, I would urge you to seek help from a family member or from someone in your diabetes team to support you in getting back on track.

8

ADJUSTING TO THE DIAGNOSIS OF TYPE 1 DIABETES

The diagnosis of type 1 diabetes strikes suddenly. It usually affects healthy children or young adults, many of whom will never have experienced significant illness at any time in their lives. Most will probably never have had to take particular notice of what they eat, nor of their levels of physical activity. And the clear majority will never have had to inject themselves with medication every day or to prick their fingers several times a day to draw blood. In many cases, literally overnight, a child or young person can transform from being a healthy and carefree person into one who for a short while becomes physically unwell, and following their recovery must face a lifetime of insulin injections and blood glucose tests, while constantly having to monitor their food intake and physical activity levels and assess their impacts on blood glucose levels. It is therefore almost to be expected that many people find it difficult to adjust to life with type 1 diabetes.

In chapter 5, I discussed some of the findings of the research undertaken by Dr Sarita Naik, who interviewed many people with type 1 diabetes about their experiences following diagnosis. Her research also explored some of the important issues that people must address following the diagnosis. She interviewed people who have lived through the diagnosis of type 1 diabetes and identified a number of key themes. It seems appropriate, therefore, to focus on these, as we discuss the importance of adjusting well to life with type 1 diabetes.

IT'S NORMAL TO BE SHOCKED AT THE DIAGNOSIS

Nearly everyone interviewed reported that receiving the diagnosis came as a shock. It was also felt that, generally, healthcare professionals had little understanding of the psychological distress associated with receiving the diagnosis and this had often been the most difficult time for individuals. Depression was a significant problem and most people felt that this had not been addressed after diagnosis or later on during their lives. One person reported: *'I thought I had the bleakest outlook on the planet. I thought my world had ended the day I was diagnosed … it is a terrible shock.'*

Shock is a natural reaction to the sudden loss of full physical health, and is the trigger to the grieving process that will often follow. You may have read about the five stages of grief. There are a number of variations but the generally-accepted five stages are denial, anger, bargaining, depression and acceptance.

One of the best accounts I have read about the stages of grief in relation to type 1 diabetes was written by Daley Kinsey on the US website, Diabetes Daily.[22] With her permission, I have reproduced her account below.

Grieving usually is associated with the death of someone or something, a dream, a loved one, a precious item. There are five stages of grieving: denial, anger, depression, bargaining, and acceptance. Everyone handles it differently. Everyone goes through the phases in some form or another, but we have to go through it to fully move on. People with diabetes usually experience these phases when they are first diagnosed. We grieve for our life of normalcy, our life before insulin injections and carb counting. In order to accept our disease and new lifestyle we have to mourn the life we used to know.

The first phase I experienced was depression. I remember when I was first diagnosed with diabetes sitting in the exam room and apologizing to my doctor because I was bawling my eyes out. Then, calling my mom and having a complete breakdown. It felt so surreal, I knew about the disease, but I didn't know anything about it. I went home and did what I usually do when I feel the world around me is out of control. I cleaned the house with tears streaming down my face. My best friend at the time came over right after I called her to comfort me; I think she may have even brought me flowers. I remember drying the dishes and telling her everything the doctor said. I felt complete guilt, how did this happen? Could I have done something different to prevent this? Why me? It was the most depressing thing for me at the time. I had just moved away from home to a new town, a new apartment, and a new life. I didn't know how I was going to handle this new condition.

Then anger set in. I remember looking at every food label for the first time. Everything had carbs in it! I was so upset; I didn't know what to eat other than water and vegetables. And at that time in my life I'd rather go hungry. Luckily I had an appointment with a nutritionist to learn how to eat as a diabetic. Once I learned how to count carbs and learned that I could still eat certain food I felt better and started to get the hang of my disease. Unfortunately, anger set in again at my next doctor's appointment. I remember being overwhelmed with information about diabetes and just snapping. I screamed at my doctor (which I feel really bad about now) that I didn't have time to be diabetic and I just needed to be fixed! Fortunately my doctor handled this outburst well and calmly explained he completely understood, and suggested attending a diabetes support group.

Bargaining was the next phase I entered. It was a short phase, but I still experienced it. I would tell myself, ok, I will take care of my diabetes as long as they promise me I won't lose my feet. When I started finger sticks I bargained with my mom that I would do them as long as I could do it on my forearm rather than on my finger. But I soon realized bargaining was not going to help my disease.

I was never in denial about having diabetes. But I was in denial that there was no cure for diabetes. I was taking a physiology class at the time and we had to do a research project on a physiological disorder. I chose to look up studies that were researching a cure for diabetes. I was hoping and praying that I would come across a groundbreaking cure and would no longer have to give myself daily injections. Unfortunately, there was no cure. I had to just come to terms with the fact that this was going to be my new lifestyle no matter how hard I tried to change that fact.

Finally, acceptance happened. It took months for it to take place, but it happened. When I accepted my new lifestyle I was able to learn everything there was to learn about it, without getting upset. I realized that I am the only person in control of my diabetes; after all it is my body that is malfunctioning. I have had my disorder for seven years and I still enter into some of these phases depending on the season of life. The nice thing is that whenever I go through a phase or two I always end up back where I need to be, accepting that this is my life and I'm ok with it.

You may relate to some of these stages, some people will relate to all of them. What is important, though, is to allow yourself to experience each stage as it arises. Do not suppress your feelings and try and ensure you do not get stuck in the intermediate stages such as denial, anger or depression and can move on to acceptance. Being able to grieve in the months after diagnosis is very important. I have seen so many examples where people have struggled with denial, anger or depression for years afterwards. The tragedy is that continuing denial can lead to a person not taking enough insulin or not paying attention to what they eat. This in turn leads to high glucose levels and all too often to the early onset of complications. Anger and resentment towards diabetes can also lead to similar outcomes. Alternatively, it can severely impact personal relationships. And depression is associated with lack of self-worth; high self-worth is essential for successful self-management of a condition such as type 1 diabetes. Put simply, you must value yourself in order to be motivated to devote adequate attention to keeping your diabetes under control. These are clear examples of where psychological issues have a very direct impact on physical health.

So, having people around you who acknowledge and share your grief is essential. It is also important to acknowledge the grief that your loved ones might also be experiencing. I can speak with some personal experience of this as when I was 25 years old, my then fiancée, Mary, was diagnosed with multiple sclerosis. In those days the complex MRI scans that today are readily available to make the diagnosis did not exist, and so it was another two years before the final diagnosis was confirmed. Adding to the difficulties in adjusting to the diagnosis was a degree of uncertainty as to what this diagnosis was, as we received different opinions from different doctors.

Nevertheless, with her first onset of symptoms, we were told quite confidently that the diagnosis was MS. Over the next few weeks I experienced a whole variety of emotions that usually expressed themselves when I was alone, as when I was with my fiancée I tried to be the strong one that helped her deal with her own thoughts and feelings, and those of the rest of the family. I found myself crying in bed at night, crying while walking the hospital corridors when on call, feeling elated at any suggestion the diagnosis could be wrong and feeling absolutely awful with any new symptom that suggested it was right. And at times I was frozen with fear at the possibility that the person I was due to marry a few months later could be stuck in a wheelchair, or worse, at any time. That fear dominated my wedding day, and came to the fore at certain key points over the next few years, such as when our children were born, or when the disease decided to strike her with another relapse.

I write this, not as a form of therapy for myself, although it probably is, but to highlight how those closest to a person with a life-changing diagnosis will have their own emotional needs that also need to be met. And while it is not your job, as someone with a new diagnosis of type 1 diabetes, to look after the needs of your partner or other loved one single-handed, my own experiences have convinced me that it is the job of the diabetes team to be aware of those needs, and where appropriate to support you together in addressing them. On many occasions, I have made a point of addressing the partner or carer of a person with type 1 diabetes very specifically to ask how they are feeling about the current situation, if they have the support they need and if there is anything that we as a team can do to help them.

In the case where a young child is diagnosed with type 1 diabetes, it is the parents who will experience a grief reaction and paediatric diabetes teams are aware to address the emotional needs of parents and other family members, as well as of the child with diabetes.

My own experiences have also convinced me of the need for open discussion, that at times might be quite painful, to enable the person with diabetes and their loved ones to express their feelings, good and bad, that arise from such a diagnosis, and to be honest in expressing if they need help to address them. I hope that understanding how your own condition can affect those around you will also help strengthen your relationships with them, long into the future.

Now while type 1 diabetes and multiple sclerosis are both autoimmune diseases that predominantly affect young people, there are very many differences. A plus for MS is that it places far less onerous self-management tasks on the individual; a minus is that there is no knowing what might happen when, and devastating disability can quickly develop. With type 1 diabetes, there is a lot that the individual can do to stabilise the condition that will help prevent nasty things happening in the future. However, neither is a nice thing to have, and both afflict previously very fit and healthy young people, who together with their loved ones, need to adjust as well as possible to life with their condition.

Just over thirty years later, we can look back and see that although Mary's condition has had its effects on both of us, by working together we have been able to adapt to those and lead a pretty normal, very happy and at times quite exciting life. That is our hope for you too.

As Daley Kinsey mentioned, in order to move on though the stages of grief, it is also important to have accurate information about diabetes, and this was also highlighted in the research conducted by Dr Naik.[23]

SUPPORT AND EDUCATION ARE IMPORTANT

The people she interviewed reported that the support and information given at diagnosis was variable and often depended on the age at which they were diagnosed. However, all individuals felt there was a lack of support and easily accessible education and this made it more difficult for them to adjust to the diagnosis. One person said: *'My initial frustration was when I first got diagnosed. I found out one day – I was in hospital and shipped out the next day with a pen and just told to inject myself. I had to see my GP to get on a training course.'*

Others reported that they received inconsistent information and that the approach used was often didactic and negative: *'The nurse came in and ripped into us about how dangerous this was and made everyone feel very down. This was counterproductive ... I remember this stunned silence.'*

It is important that the care provided by the diabetes team helps people move on from depression or denial towards acceptance. It is potentially catastrophic for such education to be given in a negative manner, that may compound any existing feelings of denial, anger, guilt or depression. Unfortunately, too often in the past, 'education' about complications has been presented as a threat, hovering over each individual if they did not 'behave' and manage their diabetes properly. All too often, 'poor control' of diabetes was associated with blame on the part of the person with diabetes, rather than on the person guiding their management or the treatment itself – again with potentially devastating consequences. I vividly remember a middle-aged man telling me that shortly after his diagnosis, some thirty years earlier, he was told by a very well-meaning nurse that if ever his blood glucose level was above 10mmol/l (180mg/dl), he should imagine a drill boring into the back of his eyes. That led him to a deep fear of high glucose levels and a tendency to run very low (and sometimes dangerously low) glucose levels for decades afterwards.

Conversely, lack of appropriate education about the action of insulin, or how to adjust insulin dose for the amount of carbohydrate eaten, can also lead to early experiences with bad hypos that can prompt a profound fear of hypos and a person running their glucose levels deliberately high for years afterwards, thus increasing their risk of complications in later life.

MEETING OTHER PEOPLE WITH DIABETES

Knowing someone else with the condition early on can help counter the impact of such events, as also highlighted by Dr Naik's research. Most of the people she interviewed did not know anyone else with type 1 diabetes. In many cases, a group education programme was the first opportunity that they had to meet and talk to other people with type 1 diabetes, and this was often many years after diagnosis. There were many benefits to meeting other people with type 1 diabetes; sharing experiences about self-management difficulties was important in helping individuals feel less isolated, particularly if they met others who had encountered similar problems. One person said: *'The first time I hardly knew anyone. At work, there were two people with type 2 diabetes. When I came to the education programme, that was the first time I had actually spoken and heard about other diabetics' goings-on – and you can say yes, that happens to you.'* And another reported that *'Coming here and actually being able to talk to people was much more useful than you would have imagined.'*

One individual felt that being able to pass on the benefit of his experiences was a positive experience not just for the recipient, but for himself as well. *'I have only just, now in the job that I am in, met two other people with diabetes. We can talk about it or talk about differences in each other's lifestyles; stuff like that is really helpful.'*

Engaging with others with type 1 diabetes early after diagnosis can help counter the isolation and withdrawal that for some people can occur during the denial or depression stages.

THE BENEFIT OF PSYCHOLOGICAL SUPPORT

Depression is a part of the grief cycle. For many this will be an understandable reaction to the perceived loss associated with the diagnosis of type 1 diabetes, and for others it could herald a more severe depression that can be difficult to shift. Dr Naik's research demonstrated that psychological support is essential to help people adjust to the diagnosis of type 1 diabetes, as well as in dealing with other issues that affected people's psychological well-being. Individuals in her study felt that there could be difficulty adjusting to erratic blood glucose levels and they did not react well to what they perceived to be less than perfect control. On the other hand, motivation to deal with intensive insulin regimes can also be hard to find. The individuals who had seen a psychologist found this support particularly helpful and felt it should be offered to all those with type 1 diabetes. However, there was recognition that not everyone would be receptive to psychological therapy. Therefore, it is important that each member of the diabetes team should have the ability to provide basic psychological support.

We introduced a psychologist to the diabetes team in Bournemouth in 1998 and many of the problems she had to deal with stemmed from issues that were unresolved from the time of diagnosis, often many years previously. In the years since then, alongside her input in addressing psychological issues with people with diabetes, an equally important part of her role has been to ensure that the whole team is aware of the need to recognise psychological issues, and provide support. I have no doubt that as a result, appropriate support provided by, for example, a diabetes nurse has helped many people deal with the psychological aspects of living with diabetes in a way that prevented these from developing into more deep-seated problems in later years.

SUPPORTIVE CLINIC VISITS

In Dr Naik's research, clinic visits were often seen to be less than satisfactory, they could be intimidating and rushed and people felt the doctor was often only interested in medical results. Consequently, some individuals often forgot about issues which they needed to talk about. Consistent with the need for appropriate psychological support, it was felt that social and personal questions should be part of the routine consultation to cover all relevant issues. This is especially important given that type 1 diabetes can affect just about every aspect of daily living.

To summarise, adjusting to the diagnosis of type 1 diabetes can be helped by your diabetes team having a real understanding of the psychological issues that arise following diagnosis, by you receiving accurate and appropriate information to help with management, by engaging with and learning from others with type 1 diabetes and by having appropriate psychological support. It is also important that clinic visits provide an opportunity for you to raise issues of concern to you.

In an ideal world, everyone will have a diabetes team that provides group support and education as well as psychological support. These are the aims of the 'Living with Diabetes' service. However, if these are not readily available to you, there are now several very good resources available online, including educational materials and discussion forums that enable you to interact with others who also have type 1 diabetes. These include:

www.bertieonline.org – an online version of the BERTIE programme that also includes a section on psychological issues.

www.diabetes.co.uk – has a lot of content relevant to this subject as well as several discussion forums that provide support from others living with type 1 diabetes.

I also hope that this book will be an ongoing source of information and support that will help address many of the issues that you might experience in the months – or years – following diagnosis.

9

THE HONEYMOON PERIOD

Type 1 diabetes occurs because the pancreas stops producing insulin. That is why a person with the condition needs treatment with insulin injections. Very often, however, once glucose levels come back to normal, and just as one begins to adapt to life with type 1 diabetes, the pancreas begins to wake up again and to start producing some insulin. This is called 'partial remission' or more commonly the 'honeymoon period'. Both terms convey something positive, and in a sense, producing insulin again should be a positive thing. However, for many people, it really does not feel much like a honeymoon, and can cause a lot of uncertainty and anxiety because of the unpredictable changes in blood glucose levels.

I have seen a number of people who have had real problems with this period. And yet it is something that I believe diabetes doctors and nurses pay too little attention to as they guide people through the important first few months of living with diabetes. The honeymoon period comes at such an important time in the life of a person with type 1 diabetes and if badly managed can leave a legacy for many years to come – thus I feel it deserves a chapter all of its own.

So, first of all, what do we know about the honeymoon period? Actually, remarkably little. A PubMed search (a sort of Google search engine for academic medical articles) came up with just 38 papers published since 1982, that is little more than one a year. This compares to over 76,000 papers on type 1 diabetes overall. What we do know is that studies suggest a honeymoon period can occur in up to 60 per cent of both adults and children with type 1 diabetes. Studies in children showed the honeymoon period started on average in the second or third month after diagnosis and lasted just under a year.[24] However, in some it lasted several years. The research showed that it was less likely to occur in children who presented with an infection, had ketoacidosis or a high HbA1c at diagnosis of type 1 diabetes. Some individuals were able to come off insulin completely during the period (complete remission) whereas in the majority of cases some insulin is still required.

It is also not fully known why a honeymoon period occurs. It is as if the pancreas is able to rest once insulin treatment has been started, and this somehow allows it to recover its ability to produce insulin again.

So, what makes the honeymoon period such a problematic time? The main reason is that there is no way of knowing when or whether the pancreas will start producing more insulin, and the first the person knows about it is that their glucose levels become much lower than usual. If this is a progressive and gradual process, this can be adapted to by reducing insulin doses. However, this in itself requires that the person recognises what is happening, and has the ability and confidence to reduce their doses themselves, or with the support of a health professional. I have seen some cases where people had no knowledge that this might happen, and continued injecting the dose of insulin prescribed by their doctor or nurse, leading to profound hypoglycaemia. Sometimes the pancreas can react very erratically, producing a surge of insulin for a short period of time. This can be very difficult to control, even in people who are able to adjust their insulin doses. In this situation, the individual needs to be supported in managing their diabetes as safely as possible until this erratic pattern subsides.

For over ten years now, the Bournemouth diabetes team has invited everyone with newly diagnosed type 1 diabetes to a group education session every three months, as described earlier. One of the unexpected benefits of attending these sessions was that people quickly learnt how to manage the effects of the honeymoon period, and as a result were able to reduce their insulin doses themselves to avoid problems. Often the first we heard about them reducing, or stopping, some insulin doses was when they came to the next session and still had stable glucose levels. That is the ideal goal of self-management education!

The following checklist on being prepared for the honeymoon period is drawn from my experience in running that programme for nearly ten years. The most important factor in being prepared for a honeymoon period is to know that it can happen, so that if it does, it does not come as a surprise. Then the following are all important:

1. Make sure you are on a basal-bolus insulin regimen. The worst problems that I have seen in a honeymoon period happened in people who were on large fixed doses of twice-daily insulin. Fortunately, that should be quite rare nowadays in the UK, but there are still some areas where this could happen. If you are in this situation, I would advise that you ask to be switched to a basal-bolus regimen as soon as possible. Not only does this more

closely mimic how the pancreas works normally, it makes it much easier to adjust your insulin doses if your pancreas does start to produce insulin again.

2. Make sure that you learn (and are taught) early on about how to adjust your basal insulin dose, and your mealtime doses. We will cover these topics in the next two chapters.

3. Make sure you have access to a specialist health professional whom you can contact if you need help with managing a honeymoon period. As I mentioned earlier, in some places there has been a tendency to leave people to their own devices once their glucose levels have settled after diagnosis. This may be appropriate for a while, but you need to know how you can quickly get back into the system if necessary.

4. Do not be afraid to reduce your insulin doses if your glucose levels start to fall for no apparent reason. If you start having hypos at night, you may need to reduce your basal insulin by a third to a half, or even more. You will not come to any harm if you cut the dose too low – yes, your glucose level will go a bit too high for a period, but that is better than having a nasty hypo because you didn't reduce the dose enough.

5. If you start having hypos after meals, reduce your mealtime dose by half. I have managed a number of people, especially those who were very active during the day, who were able to stop their breakfast and lunchtime insulin during their honeymoon period, and only have a very small dose with their evening meal.

6. During a honeymoon period, insulin requirements (especially at mealtimes) are usually very low. I would generally advise that you do not spend a lot of time working out complex insulin-to-carbohydrate ratios, nor attend an intensive self-management course, until the honeymoon period has come to an end. Not only will much of the content not apply, but once you come out of the honeymoon period, insulin requirements will quickly

increase substantially and you will have to start all over again in working out doses and ratios.

7. Finally, the honeymoon period is one example where type 1 diabetes really does try and assert itself and its control over you. Using this time to accept those parts of having diabetes that you cannot control, and learning coping mechanisms that enable you to manage those aspects that you can control, will be extremely helpful for the future.

Perhaps the best thing about the honeymoon period is that it will come to an end. This usually occurs after about a year, but it can last much longer, and in a few rare cases for many years. Perhaps another good thing about honeymoon periods is that they offer a window of opportunity when future treatments could be given to help restore normal insulin secretion, in the hope of leading to a cure. Many trials have assessed a range of possible therapies, although so far none has led to a breakthrough.

10

GETTING YOUR BASAL INSULIN DOSE RIGHT

The next few chapters will go into greater detail about how you can take control of your type 1 diabetes. However, before going any further, I would like to return to the questions I posed at the end of chapter one, repeated here:

- What are your reasons for reading this book?
- What frustrates you most about having diabetes?
- How do you want things to be different?
- How will you know when you have achieved this?
- What is the main thing you would like to change after reading this book?

It may be that the answers you wrote at the beginning still apply. However, it could also be that your goals have changed somewhat, having read the first few chapters. If so, take a few minutes to update them. Perhaps you are not yet sure on what your main goals will be? Never mind, read on – we will look at these questions again in chapter 22.

This chapter aims to support you in ensuring that you are taking the right amount of basal insulin. It is designed for people on multiple daily injections of insulin, including one or two injections each day of basal insulin. The basic principles are similar for people on an insulin pump, although a pump does allow for more detailed fine-tuning of the basal dose (described in more detail in chapter 13). If you do use an insulin pump though, I would still recommend that you read this chapter to ensure you understand the principles underlying the role of basal insulin.

As discussed earlier, there are a number of different types of insulin that are used for basal insulin. These are in two main categories: isophane or analogue insulin. Isophane insulins are traditional basal insulins; they are manufactured using human insulin (produced by specially programmed bacteria) that is in a suspension to slow down its absorption, so that its effect lasts many hours. These insulins were typically used once a day. The main problem with them is that absorption from the injection site could be very erratic and lead to unpredictable glucose levels, especially overnight. This was compounded by the fact that these insulins had a peak effect a few hours after injection and so some people would need to have a carbohydrate-containing snack to avoid hypoglycaemia. Sometimes this could be overcome by using a smaller dose twice daily, but the erratic absorption and peak level would still be there, although somewhat less marked.

In my opinion, one of the greatest advances in management of type 1 diabetes in the last 20 years came with the arrival of the first long-acting insulin analogue: glargine, marketed by Sanofi as Lantus™. An insulin analogue is produced by manufacturing human insulin with a slight change in its chemical structure to make it stick together to be released slowly into the bloodstream. The arrival of Lantus was in many ways a quiet revolution in the management of type 1 diabetes and many people who switched from older insulins to Lantus noticed an almost immediate improvement. The most common feedback that I had was that it brought about stable blood glucose levels, particularly overnight, so that people became more confident in going to bed with a good glucose level without worrying that they could have a hypo during the night. Remember that the older insulins could be very variable in how they were absorbed, meaning that some nights a dose could work well, but on others the same dose could lead to a high level by morning, or even worse a bad hypo during the night. Because of this, many people were advised to have a snack at bedtime in case their insulin would otherwise cause a hypo. The problem then of course is that the snack would often push glucose levels up too high by the next morning.

The introduction of Lantus led to further benefits in our ability to control glucose levels at night. Given that it was much better at keeping glucose levels stable, this meant that people could be more confident about going to bed with a near-normal blood glucose level, and not worry that it would go too low overnight. Before long, we started advising that people could use a correction dose of fast-acting insulin at bedtime if their glucose level was too high. So, in a space of a few years, we switched from advising a bedtime snack (with no insulin to cover it) to advising a bedtime correction dose of fast-acting insulin (with no carbohydrate to cover it) – quite a change! If you are still in the habit of taking a snack at bedtime, then I can understand that changing that habit to taking extra insulin at bedtime with no snack will not be easy. It should be done in a number of steps, preferably with the support of a diabetes doctor or educator, to help you gain confidence that it is safe. This particularly applies if you are still using an older isophane insulin

However, there were downsides that came with Lantus too. The biggest in my view was that it was very heavily marketed for use in type 2 diabetes, backed up by trials that appeared to show it was very good at controlling type 2 diabetes with just one injection a day, and with just one blood test each morning. It was claimed to be so easy that non-specialists could use Lantus to control type 2 diabetes, all they had to do was keep increasing the dose until the fasting glucose level was normal. Fifteen years, and many billions in sales later, it is evident that Lantus is no better than the older insulins for type 2 diabetes. More worryingly, the notion that you keep increasing the dose based on one blood test a day rather misses important points about the ideal management of type 2 diabetes, namely what happens to glucose levels later during the day. We didn't know because they weren't checked, but in most cases, as people ate during the day their glucose levels will have risen to quite high levels by bedtime, requiring a high dose of Lantus to bring the glucose level down overnight. Most worryingly, the same strategy seeped through into how Lantus was used in type 1 diabetes, with at times catastrophic results with hypos. It also completely diverted attention away from how a basal insulin should be used, that is to keep glucose levels stable and not as a tool to correct high levels.

There are now other brands of glargine (the generic name for Lantus), such as Abasaglar™ (or Basaglar™ in US), marketed by Lilly. In addition to glargine, there are also other long-acting analogues available. The first is Levemir™ (detemir), produced by Novo Nordisk. This has a shorter action than Lantus and needs to be given twice a day. Unfortunately, however, it was launched as an insulin that could be given once a day (presumably to compete with Lantus) and so again the marketing of a product led to suboptimal treatment in many people, in whom quite simply the insulin ran out during the day. Ironically Levemir is actually very good when used twice a day as will be discussed in more detail later in this chapter.

The third analogue is Tresiba™ (degludec), also manufactured by Novo Nordisk. This is longer acting than Levemir and Lantus, and the early data suggested it could be given every 2 to 3 days. In fact, it needs to be given once a day, and could be an alternative for those in whom Lantus does not last the whole day.

So, how do you get the basal level right? I will start by describing how I recommend this is done using Lantus, before discussing using the alternatives.

ONCE DAILY BASAL INSULIN

At diagnosis, it is customary to start on a modest dose of Lantus at bedtime, say 10 units. As glucose levels are usually high at this time, Lantus is used to help bring glucose levels down gradually over a period of one to two weeks. Thus, if after the first three days it is clear that levels are not falling, then the dose will need to be increased. As glucose levels fall towards normal levels (for example 5–7mmol/l (90–120mg/dl)) in the morning, when fasting, then the dose of Lantus should be reviewed and adjusted if required, until the dose is found that keeps glucose levels stable overnight. These initial adjustments are best done with the support of a health professional with experience and expertise in managing diabetes.

Note that the key is to find the dose of Lantus that keeps glucose levels *stable* overnight, not the one that achieves a normal fasting blood glucose. So, at this stage, if the blood glucose is 10mmol/l (180mg/dl) at bedtime, the right dose of Lantus is the one that keeps the level stable overnight, so that the level in the morning is also 10mmol/l (180mg/dl), even though both are too high.

Unfortunately, I still come across people who have been told that the right dose of Lantus is the dose that will bring a bedtime blood glucose level of 10mmol/l (180mg/dl) down to 5mmol/l (90mg/dl) the next morning. I suspect that the guidance that was circulated about using Lantus when it was launched has played a role in perpetuating such advice for people with type 1 diabetes, even though the guidance was designed for treatment of people with type 2 diabetes. While this might work in the short term, what will happen if one night your glucose level is only 7mmol/l (120mg/dl)? You will of course go hypo during the night. It is also important to note that Lantus (or any other basal insulin) cannot be changed on a daily basis according to the bedtime glucose level. As it is so long acting, not only will any change affect glucose levels overnight, it will also affect them for most of the next day too. It is more of a strategic player, and once the right dose has been identified, this same dose should be used each day. And while adjusting to find the right dose, as it is so long-acting, it is important to wait at least three days before changing the dose.

Once you have found the correct dose, you can work on getting your bedtime blood glucose level down to normal (for example 5–7mmol/l (90–120mg/dl)) in the knowledge that the same dose of Lantus will keep it at that level until the next morning. Achieving a normal bedtime level will require adjustment of the rapid-acting insulin taken with the evening meal, and possibly a correction dose of the same insulin at bedtime. This will be covered in the next chapter.

The following examples show what this means in practice. Each example shows a blood glucose diary over a few days. Have a look and decide whether the basal insulin dose needs changing.

Example 1. Sam was diagnosed with type 1 diabetes four months ago. He now takes 18 units of Lantus at bedtime. His morning glucose levels are high.

		Before breakfast	Before lunch	Before evening meal	Before bed
Day 1	mmol/l	9.8	7.9	10.3	7.4
	mg/dl	176	142	185	133
Day 2	mmol/l	10.1	8.4	7.5	7.1
	mg/dl	182	151	135	128
Day 3	mmol/l	11.2	5.6	8.4	8.1
	mg/dl	202	101	151	146

In this case, the morning levels are higher than the night before. Therefore, the basal insulin is not doing its job in keeping levels stable overnight. He could try increasing the dose to 20 units.

Example 2. Sara has had type 1 diabetes for eight months. She has had some hypos in the night and has reduced her Lantus from 20 to 16 units. This has stopped the hypos, and she is quite happy with her morning levels now.

		Before breakfast	Before lunch	Before evening meal	Before bed
Day 1	mmol/l	5.6	6.5	6.9	9.2
	mg/dl	101	117	124	166
Day 2	mmol/l	4.8	5.3	7.9	11.1
	mg/dl	86	95	142	200
Day 3	mmol/l	5.2	4.5	5.6	8.5
	mg/dl	94	81	101	153

Her glucose levels in the morning are within the normal range, but they are a lot lower than the night before, meaning that the basal insulin is pulling her glucose level down overnight. Although she is no longer waking up with a hypo during the night, she is at risk of having one. Look at her glucose level at bedtime on the third day. It is 8.5mmol/l (153mg/dl), and if it was to drop by 5.9mmol/l

(106mg/dl) overnight, as on the second day, then her level will fall to less than 3mmol/l (54mg/dl) or even lower. She needs to reduce her Lantus, maybe to 12 units to prevent this happening.

Example 3. Sara has reduced her basal insulin but she now thinks her morning levels are too high

		Before breakfast	Before lunch	Before evening meal	Before bed
Day 1	mmol/l	8.4	6.8	5.4	9.2
	mg/dl	151	122	97	166
Day 2	mmol/l	9.0	7.2	7.8	10.3
	mg/dl	162	130	140	185
Day 3	mmol/l	11.4	8.9	7.9	8.9
	mg/dl	205	160	142	160

Although the morning levels are high, they are quite similar to the readings the night before. Therefore, she is on the right dose of basal insulin and this does not need to change. The problem is that her glucose levels rise after her evening meal – so she would benefit by having more insulin (or less carbohydrate) with her evening meal, to keep her glucose at a more reasonable level at bedtime. This will be discussed in the next chapter.

Checking the basal insulin during the day

So far, we have looked at what happens at night in determining whether the dose of basal insulin is correct. But basal insulin needs to keep the glucose level stable through the day and the night. Look back at the last example, where the levels are going up in the evening. Supposing Sara said that on the first two evenings she had a meal with no carbohydrate and thus she didn't take any insulin for it. In this case, a likely reason for the glucose level rising is that the Lantus is beginning to run out, and so it is unable to keep the glucose level stable.

If you find that your glucose levels are fine overnight but then tend to rise sometime during the day, it would be worth doing a specific check to see whether the basal insulin is keeping levels stable. The best way of doing this is a so-called 'fasting profile'. Essentially this means missing a meal (or having a carbohydrate-free meal) and watching what happens to the glucose level over the next few hours. If you take your basal insulin at bedtime, then it is likely that the dose will run out sometime during the next afternoon, at the earliest. So, to test this, you would need to see what happens to your glucose level with no carbohydrates or fast-acting insulin on board from midday onwards. This is best done in two separate steps, so on one day you could miss lunch, and on another day, miss (or delay) your evening meal, as follows:

Day 1: Check your glucose first thing in the morning and have breakfast as normal, ideally before 9am. After that you should not eat or drink any carbohydrate until your evening meal. You can drink black tea or coffee or water and have a carbohydrate-free snack or meal at lunchtime. Check your glucose level at about midday, then at 3pm and then just before your evening meal, ideally around 6-7pm. This should be a normal meal (with carbohydrate if you want) and your normal mealtime insulin. The aim is that the glucose level should be about the same at each time point (12 noon, 3pm and 6pm).

Day 2: Check your glucose first thing in the morning and have breakfast as normal, ideally before 9am. After that you can eat and drink normally and have your usual lunch, with mealtime insulin, ideally between 12 and 1pm. After that you should not eat or drink any carbohydrate until after 9pm. You can drink black tea or coffee or water and have a carbohydrate-free snack at tea time. Check your glucose level at about 3pm, 6pm and 9pm. You can then have a late meal which should be a normal meal (with carbohydrate if you want) and your normal mealtime insulin. You can chart the fasting periods as below. The aim is that the glucose level should be about the same at each time point (3pm, 6pm and 9pm).

	12noon	3pm	6pm	9pm
Day 1				
Day 2				

If the basal insulin runs out in the evening, your results will look something like this:

		12noon	3pm	6pm	9pm
Day 1	mmol/l	6.3	6.8	7.1	
	mg/dl	113	122	128	
Day 2	mmol/l		6.7	7.3	9.1
	mg/dl		121	131	164

As there is reasonable control until 6pm, you can probably manage with just the night time injection of basal insulin, as long as you are aware that if you delay your evening meal, your glucose levels may begin to rise in the early evening. This can be corrected using your mealtime insulin, as we will discuss in the next chapter.

If your basal insulin runs out in the early afternoon, then you will get something like this:

		12noon	3pm	6pm	9pm
Day 1	mmol/l	6.2	8.6	11.3	
	mg/dl	112	155	203	
Day 2	mmol/l		6.8	9.6	12.3
	mg/dl		122	173	221

In this situation, you really need to have a second injection of basal insulin in the morning, as covered in the next section.

Once daily injections of other basal insulins

I would not recommend Levemir as a once-daily basal insulin as I have found that in many people, it just does not last long enough. If you are on once daily Levemir, then the best option is probably to add a second dose of Levemir to provide full 24-hour coverage. If you are not happy about taking an extra injection, then switching to Lantus or Degludec would be appropriate.

In some countries, analogue insulins are either not available or are too expensive for many people to use. In these situations, NPH or isophane versions of human insulin (for example Insulatard or Humulin I) can be used as the basal insulin. In view of the possible problems associated with these insulins due to their shorter action and more erratic absorption, I would recommend these are used twice daily, as described below, rather than once daily.

Degludec is a new long-acting analogue to come on the market. Studies suggest it is similar to Lantus, but at higher cost. In the UK, the cost has come down but in some areas it can only be prescribed by a diabetes specialist. It is an option for people where Lantus does not cover the whole 24-hour period but who do not wish to split the dose, or in those in which it is difficult to avoid hypos at night with Lantus.

SPLIT BASAL DOSE – TWO INJECTIONS A DAY

The 2015 UK NICE guidelines recommend that twice-daily Levemir should be used as the preferred basal insulin in type 1 diabetes, as there is some evidence that it provides for better control than once-daily Lantus.[25] However, many centres still recommend once-daily Lantus to start with, and this does seem reasonable, especially if it provides stable control on one injection.

Twice-daily Lantus

If you are on once-daily Lantus, and your testing reveals that it is not sufficient in providing 24-hour cover, then you have two options. To add a second dose of Lantus, or to switch to twice-daily Levemir.

Adding a second dose of Lantus has the advantage that you do not need to change the type of insulin and in most cases this is what I would recommend at first. If your current dose of Lantus keeps your glucose stable overnight, but glucose levels then rise later in the day, then I would suggest staying on the same dose of Lantus at bedtime, and adding a small dose in the morning, to be taken before breakfast. This could start at no more than 4 units, and can be adjusted after a few days if necessary. If, however, your current dose of Lantus causes your glucose level to fall overnight, and it then rises during the day, then I would decrease the evening dose of Lantus by the same amount as the second dose to be introduced in the morning. Quite how much will depend on your particular circumstances, and I advise that you seek the support of your diabetes team in deciding on the optimal change in dose.

The main disadvantage of using a split dose of Lantus is that, as it is quite a long-acting insulin, the doses could overlap and theoretically increase the risk of a hypo, especially during the morning. In my experience, this is less of a problem in reality, as long as one starts with a low dose in the mornings. However, for people who are very active during the day, it may be preferable to switch to Levemir, which is shorter acting and with less risk of the doses overlapping.

Twice-daily Levemir

The shorter action of Levemir gives it a good advantage when used as a twice-daily basal insulin, as there is less risk that the doses will overlap. For this reason, it is likely that the doses will need to be more evenly divided than with Lantus. As an example, a typical dose of Levemir could be 8 units in the morning and 12 units at night (rather than 4 and 16 respectively for Lantus). Again, I recommend consulting with your diabetes team for advice on exact doses. The same principle applies, namely that the night-time dose should keep the glucose level stable overnight, and so is best assessed by comparing the blood glucose level at bedtime and the next morning. The morning dose should keep the glucose level stable through the day. This can be assessed in the same way as described above for Lantus, by checking glucose levels on a day when you fast (or have no carbohydrate) at lunchtime and on another day when you 'fast' in the evening.

The shorter action of Levemir also gives more flexibility in being able to adjust the dose, to take into account different levels of physical activity. This is especially useful for people who play sport or engage in other forms of prolonged activity. On a day of such activity, a lower dose of Levemir can be taken in the morning to reduce the risk of a hypo, without affecting the control overnight. This is not possible in the same way with a longer-acting insulin such as Lantus. This is illustrated in the following example:

Katherine enjoys long-distance running. At weekends, she runs for up to 20km a day, usually starting around ten o'clock on a Sunday morning. During the week she runs shorter distances in the evenings. She takes twice daily Levemir, at a usual dose of 12 units at bedtime and 8 units in the morning. On the morning before a long run, she reduces her Levemir to 4 units. This enables her to run without the worry of hypoglycaemia.

Twice-daily NPH insulin

For many years, these were the only insulins available as a basal insulin and, as discussed earlier, in many countries they have been replaced by the newer analogue insulins. However, for some people, older NPH or isophane insulins are the only available option, and so they are included here. The main NPH insulins available are Insulatard (Novo Nordisk), Humulin I (Lilly) and Insuman Basal (Sanofi). I recommend they are used twice a day, in the same way as described above for Levemir. However, one has to be careful of the increased risk of a hypo a few hours after injection, due to the peak action at that time. Thus, it might make sense to have the evening dose in the early evening (perhaps with the evening meal, at the same time as the mealtime insulin but as a separate injection), rather than at bedtime. Having a meal afterwards will reduce the risk of a hypo, and the earlier injection time means that it will be possible to check the glucose before bed to make sure the level is not too low. NPH insulins do not produce the same stable blood glucose profile as more modern analogues, and so it can be less easy to establish the correct dose than when using analogue insulin. However, it should be possible to use overnight glucose values to determine the best dose of NPH to take in the evening, as in the following examples:

Dan takes NPH insulin with breakfast (8 units) and with his evening meal (12 units). His glucose values over three days are as shown below.

		Before breakfast	Before lunch	Before evening meal	Before bed
Day 1	mmol/l	8.4	6.8	7.8	6.5
	mg/dl	151	122	140	117
Day 2	mmol/l	9.0	7.2	7.8	5.9
	mg/dl	162	130	140	106
Day 3	mmol/l	6.4	8.9	7.9	6.1
	mg/dl	115	160	142	110

Note that on day 1, his level dropped by bedtime but then rose again overnight. This could represent the 'peak' effect of NPH a few hours after injection causing the lower value at bedtime, and then the insulin's effect lessening overnight.

Increasing the evening dose of NPH could risk the glucose level falling too low at bedtime. Note that on day 3, the morning glucose value is also quite low (although in the normal range) and so increasing the dose could result in a hypo during the night from day 2 to day 3. Avoiding hypos is the top priority and so it is preferable to keep the same dose of NPH and if the glucose is high in the morning, to take a slightly higher dose of mealtime insulin with breakfast to bring the glucose level down again.

Daniela also takes NPH twice daily, 10 units in the morning and 16 units with her evening meal. Her readings are generally quite high overnight:

		Before breakfast	Before lunch	Before evening meal	Before bed
Day 1	mmol/l	10.1	7.1	6.9	8.1
	mg/dl	182	128	124	146
Day 2	mmol/l	11.1	8.2	7.8	8.7
	mg/dl	200	148	140	157
Day 3	mmol/l	9.5	8.7	8.9	9.1
	mg/dl	171	157	160	164

Her glucose levels increase from the time of her evening meal to bedtime and then also increase further overnight. In this situation, it is reasonable to increase the evening dose of NPH, with the aim of achieving bedtime levels of around 6–7mmol/l (110–130mg/dl). In such a case, a small increase say of 2 units may well be enough. As with the previous case, any rise overnight can be corrected when necessary with some extra mealtime insulin with breakfast.

David has the opposite problem. He takes 12 units in the morning and 18 in the evening. His glucose levels tend to fall overnight:

		Before breakfast	Before lunch	Before evening meal	Before bed
Day 1	mmol/l	5.6	7.1	7.8	8.1
	mg/dl	101	128	140	146
Day 2	mmol/l	4.3	7.9	8.6	8.5
	mg/dl	77	142	155	153
Day 3	mmol/l	6.5	8.7	8.9	8.8
	mg/dl	117	157	160	158

As with analogue insulin, the aim of NPH insulin should be to keep glucose levels stable overnight. When levels fall overnight there is always an increased risk of a hypo during the night and so the recommendation is to reduce the evening dose of NPH, initially by 2 units, until the morning levels are about the same as at bedtime. This is harder to achieve with NPH than with analogue insulin but at least one should aim to avoid a general trend of levels falling overnight. Once this has been achieved, he may need to take a bit more mealtime insulin in the evening to bring the bedtime glucose levels down to a more reasonable level, for example between 6 and 8mmol/l or 120–140mg/dl.

Performing a fasting profile during the day (by missing breakfast or lunch for example or having a carbohydrate-free meal, as described on page 123) could increase the risk of hypoglycaemia because of the increased action of the insulin a few hours after injection, and is therefore not generally advised. Rather, it is safer to use routine blood glucose testing before meals to determine that the dose of NPH insulin is about right. This can be assessed by observing any change in glucose levels between breakfast and lunch, and between lunch and the evening meal. For a dose of

NPH taken with breakfast, the greatest risk of a hypo is between breakfast and lunch, and so it is important to ensure glucose levels do not fall between these times. After lunch is the time when the dose may begin to run out, and this would be indicated by a tendency for glucose levels to rise before the evening meal, as shown in the following example.

Joao takes 12 units of NPH insulin with breakfast and 16 units with his evening meal. He sometimes experiences mild hypos before lunch.

	Before breakfast	Before lunch	Before evening meal	Before bed
mmol/l	8.4	3.9	8.6	9.2
mg/dl	151	70	155	166
mmol/l	8.8	4.6	7.8	10.3
mg/dl	158	83	140	185
mmol/l	9.7	4.1	7.9	8.9
mg/dl	175	74	142	160

In this example, it can be seen that his glucose levels remain quite stable overnight, suggesting that the evening dose of NPH is about right. However, levels drop before lunch and then rise again before the evening meal. This reflects the peak action of the morning dose before lunch, and that the insulin's effect is likely to be wearing off in the afternoon. In this situation, increasing the dose to improve the afternoon cover will increase the risk of a hypo before lunch. On the other hand, reducing the dose to reduce the risk of a hypo will lead to higher glucose levels in the afternoon. Thus, the best way of addressing this is likely to be by making slight changes to the mealtime insulin. A slightly lower dose with breakfast should offset the tendency to go low before lunch, and a slightly higher dose at lunchtime should make up for the waning effect of the NPH in the afternoon. This will be covered in more detail in the next chapter.

11

CALCULATING MEALTIME (BOLUS) INSULIN DOSES

In the late 1980s, when I first started working in diabetes, many people with type 1 diabetes were on two injections a day of mixed insulin, such as Mixtard (that contained 30 per cent short-acting and 70 per cent intermediate-acting insulin). Theoretically they were also provided with a diet 'prescription' that set out the grams of carbohydrate they should eat with each meal every day, that looked something like this:

Breakfast	60g
Morning snack	20g
Lunch	60g
Afternoon snack	20g
Evening meal	80g

Bedtime snack	20g
Total	260g

Note how snacks were included in this prescription. This is because the insulins in the injections would have led to quite high blood insulin levels in the day, and without the snacks there was a risk of the individual having a hypo. The bedtime snack was also designed to protect from a hypo during the night. Note also that the total carbohydrate intake was quite high, usually between two and three hundred grams a day, which is the recommended intake for the general population.

In practice, while many did see a dietitian at times, I was aware that there was not always enough time to explain how to count carbohydrates, and as a result, the amount eaten each day could vary quite considerably, while the insulin dose was fixed to be the same every day. It was the job of the doctor to adjust the insulin dose at clinic visits. It is hardly surprising, therefore, that many people experienced big swings in the blood glucose levels, that sometimes, as in the case of the person I mentioned in chapter 3, came to dominate their lives.

The first insulin pen was produced by Novo in 1985. It was called the NovoPen and started a transformation in the way type 1 diabetes was managed, as it was the NovoPen that introduced most of the world to the basal bolus regimen that we now regard as standard practice for type 1 diabetes. At that time, it was called the 'NovoPen regimen'. It introduced the concept of mealtime insulin, separate from the basal insulin. At that time, the only insulins available were the newly-introduced 'human' insulins (actually produced by genetically modified bacteria). The NovoPen dispensed the Novo version, called Actrapid. In fact, by today's standards it was anything but rapid, taking up to two hours to reach peak effect and then lasting for up to seven or eight hours. Thus, it had to be injected at least 30 minutes before a meal, and the meal usually had to be followed by a snack two hours later to avoid the risk of hypoglycaemia. However, it was a start, and as a separate injection was given for each meal, it provided freedom to vary the time of meals and to vary the amount eaten, as the dose could be altered from meal to meal. The first NovoPen had a button at the end that dispensed two units for each press of the button. A dose of ten units required five presses. Although the dose could be altered, in practice (in the UK at least) people were prescribed a standard dose for each meal. Commonly this would be about 8 to 10 units.

By the early 1990s, the idea of 'carbohydrate prescriptions' had been abandoned, as a policy paper from the British Diabetic Association (now known as Diabetes UK), stated that what was important was that people with diabetes should eat healthily rather than count their carbohydrates.[25] And so anyone diagnosed with type 1 diabetes from about 1992 was provided with next to no information about what foods had carbohydrates in them or how to count them. Rather they were just told to eat a healthy diet, and inject a prescribed dose of insulin before each meal. So, although the advent of the NovoPen brought the potential for matching insulin doses to the carbohydrate eaten, in practice this did not happen, and people still suffered the same fluctuations in their glucose levels.

In 1993, I started work at St Thomas' Hospital in London, right opposite Big Ben and the Houses of Parliament. St Thomas' Hospital has a long and proud history, home to many medical advances since it was founded in 1173. It was also where Florence Nightingale founded the world's first modern school of nursing. I worked for three years in the department of Diabetes under Professor Peter Sonksen, who in the 1970s was involved in the development of the world's first home blood glucose meters. He also was one of the pioneers of the current method for treating diabetic ketoacidosis. Shortly before I started there, he called me and said he would like me to work on a computer system that would help people with type 1 diabetes work out their insulin doses. It sounded a crazy idea to me, but I didn't feel it was a good idea to say no to a highly-regarded Professor before I had even started the job. And so started my involvement with the Diabetes Insulin Advisory System (or DIAS for short), a complex computer model developed by clever mathematicians in London and Denmark that aimed to predict what happened to glucose levels during the day and night, between the four or five measurements taken using home blood testing. In the three years that I worked at St Thomas', and for some time afterwards, I was involved in several projects that tested the DIAS system. From this I learnt a number of key lessons that were to transform my approach to the management of type 1 diabetes:

1. Blood glucose levels rise, and thus the amount of insulin required increases, according to the amount of carbohydrate eaten. This seems a no-brainer now, but at the time, there was little concept of adjusting insulin according to carbohydrate intake.

2. It is possible to have a profound hypo between two normal blood glucose readings, a few hours apart. Thus, if the reading was 6.1mmol/l (110mg/dl) before breakfast and 7.8mmol/l (140mg/dl) before lunch, the glucose level didn't necessarily gradually rise during the morning, but could well have fallen steeply to 2.5mmol/l (45mg/dl) mid-morning. This was particularly likely to happen using the older short-acting insulins in use then, as the dose taken at breakfast would still have been very active 2–3 hours after the meal.

3. Often these hypos were very frequent and unrecognised as a result of loss of hypo warning signs (hypoglycaemic unawareness, as discussed in chapter 3).

4. Hypos during the night were also quite common, and followed by very high glucose values the next day. This so-called 'Somogyi phenomenon' was first described by a Hungarian Physician, Dr Somogyi, in the 1930s.[26] It is thought that the stress hormones released in response to the hypo then cause the glucose levels to rise. Many people with diabetes will have experienced this phenomenon, although many experts dispute it, as it has been very hard to prove its existence in research studies. However, I am a firm believer as I have seen several cases where reducing the night-time insulin led to lower insulin levels the next morning. The only way I can explain that is that the reduced insulin avoided a hypo, that in turn avoided the rebound high glucose levels the next day. In those early DIAS studies, we also saw cases where individuals struggled with glucose levels that varied from very low to very high on almost a daily basis. On the principle that the highs were often a result of the lows, we focused on reducing insulin doses to avoid the lows, and this in turn prevented the rebound highs. As a result, we saw several cases where the average measured blood glucose levels improved after significantly reducing the insulin dose – the opposite to what you would normally expect.

Taken together, the lessons learnt from this research were that:

- mealtime insulin needs to be adjusted according to the carbohydrate content of the meal;
- in many cases, standard insulin doses were too high and needed to be reduced;
- when glucose levels fluctuate, the priority is to reduce insulin to avoid the hypos as the high glucose levels will then often 'sort themselves out'.

When I moved to Bournemouth to take up my post as a Consultant in 1996, I continued to work on DIAS for a few years, using it to help guide people with poorly-controlled diabetes in achieving more stable control. They often shared several common themes: they knew very little about which foods contained carbohydrates and therefore they did not know how to adjust mealtime insulin doses. They also had little knowledge of how to treat a hypo (often giving themselves much too much glucose – another cause of high levels following a hypo), nor did they understand the effect of exercise or other factors on their insulin requirements. It was not their fault that they didn't know these key pieces of information, it was just that they hadn't been effectively taught – and in too many cases just hadn't been told these things at all.

DIAS was eventually superseded by the advent of continuous glucose monitoring systems in the early 2000s, but the lessons learnt from its use led directly to the development of BERTIE, the Bournemouth type 1 intensive education programme, that was first piloted in 1998, and has been running ever since, not only in Bournemouth, but also in many other diabetes centres across the UK, who were trained by the Bournemouth team in implementing locally-adapted versions of BERTIE.

BERTIE is a course that consists of four day-long sessions at weekly intervals, to train people with type 1 diabetes in carbohydrate counting and insulin dose adjustment. I would strongly recommend anyone who has not done so to attend such a course, so that they can learn from local experts about how to use their insulin doses to achieve stable control of their diabetes. For those who cannot access such a course, then an online version, available at www.bertieonline. org.uk is a good second best, providing the key content via an e-learning platform. It is accessible free of charge from anywhere in the world. The *Carbs & Cals* book and app provide an extremely useful resource to help people assess the amount of carbohydrate in different portion sizes of many foods, which is of course essential in calculating how much insulin to give. There are US and UK versions available.

The next section provides a detailed account of the principles that underpin the approach covered in BERTIE. These apply equally to those using insulin pens or syringes as well as those using insulin pumps.

INSULIN TO CARBOHYDRATE RATIO (ICR)

Any rapid-acting insulin analogue will be sufficient for most people's needs. Commonly used analogues include lispro (Humalog™), aspart (Novorapid™ or Novolog™) and glulisine (Apidra™). Recently an even faster-acting version of aspart has been marketed under the name of Fiasp™. In areas where these are not available or are too expensive, short-acting human insulin (for example Actrapid™ or Humulin S™, or Humulin R™ in the US) can be used, although care needs to be taken in view of its longer duration of action.

When using carbohydrate counting to determine your mealtime insulin doses, the idea is that you do not have a set dose for each meal, but rather that you use your ICR to work out how much insulin you need for the carbohydrate in the meal you are about to eat. In Chapter 5, I advised that a good starting point is to use an ICR of 1 unit of insulin for every 10 grams of carbohydrate, unless the total insulin dose (including basal insulin) is less than 30 units a day, in which case half a unit should be enough for every 10 grams of carbohydrate.

When starting out, I generally advise to use the same ICR for all meals, unless your activity level is very different at different times of day. For example, someone who has a very physical job such as a labourer on a building site, may find they need much less insulin during the working day (so need a lower dose at breakfast and at lunchtime), than in the evening. Alternatively, someone who sits at a computer all day but then plays sport in the evening will need relatively more insulin at breakfast and at lunch than in the evening. In these situations, you could start out as follows:

	Breakfast	Lunch	Evening meal
Equally active all day	1 unit per 10g	1 unit per 10g	1 unit per 10g
More active in the day; less active in the evening	0.5 unit per 10g	0.5 unit per 10g	1 unit per 10g
Less active in the day; more active in the evening	1 unit per 10g	1 unit per 10g	0.5 unit per 10g

Any insulin given for snacks in the morning or afternoon would use the daytime ICR to calculate the dose; snacks after the evening meal would use the evening ICR. However, if a dose is given within three hours of the previous insulin dose, then some of that dose will still be active (so-called 'insulin on board') and a slightly smaller dose will be needed. For this reason, initially at least, I would suggest not injecting any insulin for a snack of 20g of carbohydrate or less.

As long as you check your blood glucose each time you inject, you will soon begin to see if your ICR is working well for you. Generally, if it is, then the next glucose level after the meal should be about the same as the one before the meal, as in the following example:

		Breakfast	Lunch	Evening meal	Bedtime
Day 1	mmol/l	6.1	6.9	7.1	7.3
	mg/dl	110	124	128	131
Day 2	mmol/l	6.8	6.4	6.1	6.8
	mg/dl	122	115	110	122
Day 3	mmol/l	6.4	6.8	7.1	5.9
	mg/dl	115	122	128	106

However, if the next reading is higher than the previous one, then a higher ICR will be necessary:

		Breakfast	Lunch	Evening meal	Bedtime
Day 1	mmol/l	6.1	8.9	10.1	10.9
	mg/dl	110	160	182	196
Day 2	mmol/l	10.7	11.3	12.1	11.0
	mg/dl	193	203	218	198
Day 3	mmol/l	12.0	12.8	13.8	15.0
	mg/dl	216	230	248	270

In this case, each reading is higher than the previous one, suggesting that for every meal, more insulin was required. And so instead of an ICR of 1, then an ICR of 1.5 units per 10g of carbohydrate might be needed.

Sometimes, you will see a different response for different times of day:

		Breakfast	Lunch	Evening meal	Bedtime
Day 1	mmol/l	6.1	8.9	8.7	7.8
	mg/dl	110	160	157	140
Day 2	mmol/l	7.5	10.1	9.1	8.9
	mg/dl	135	182	164	160
Day 3	mmol/l	8.0	10.6	10.5	9.9
	mg/dl	144	191	189	178

In this last example, the glucose level rises by up to 3mmol/l or 50mg/dl between breakfast and lunch, but is reasonably stable for the rest of the day. This would suggest a higher ICR is needed with breakfast than with the other meals. This is quite a common finding, as a result of the various hormones such as cortisol and growth hormone that are at high levels in the early morning, and that make insulin less effective (so you need to inject more). Note than in the last example, the glucose levels tended to drop a little by bedtime. The important thing is to correct the biggest issue (i.e. a higher ICR in the morning) first of all. Once this has been done, it might be necessary to reduce the ICR with the evening meal.

I generally express the ICR as units of insulin required per 10g of carbohydrate. The alternative way of describing the same thing is to say how many grams of carbohydrate require one unit of insulin, which is a bit like using MPG (miles per gallon) to express how much fuel your car needs. In Germany and other countries, the same concept is expressed by saying how many litres of fuel are required to drive 100 kilometres (or how many gallons to drive 100 miles to use US terms). This is the equivalent to units per 10g of carbohydrate.

To explain this a little further, if you use 1 unit per 10g of carbohydrate and find that this is not enough, you either need to have more insulin for the same amount of carbohydrate (i.e. 1.5 units per 10g), or less carbohydrate for that one unit of insulin (1 unit per 7g). They are just two different ways of saying the same thing. I prefer the former – units per 10g of carbohydrate – as I think the maths is easier. You just have to work out how many grams of carbohydrate are in your meal, multiply by your ICR then divide by 10 then. So, if you are about to eat a meal with 40g of carbohydrate, and you have 1.5 units per 10g, then the dose you need is:

40 x 1.5 ÷ 10 = 6 units

If your ratio is 1 unit per 10g of carbohydrate it is even easier:

40 x 1÷ 10, or 40 ÷ 10 = 4

On the other hand, if you have 1 unit per 7g of carbohydrate, you need to divide your meal (40g) by 7 to get 6 (or thereabouts).

This requires you to be able to divide by whatever your ICR is; for many people this is more difficult than multiplication. At the end of the day, it doesn't really matter which system you use, as long as you are consistent in using one system and you are confident how to use it.

Once you have your ICR, you need to know how to add up all the carbohydrate in the meal you are about to eat. Remember that all starchy foods contain carbohydrate, such as bread, potatoes, pasta, rice and other grains and cereals. And anything with sugar. Sweet foods are relatively easy to identify, but don't forget that many processed foods and many sauces and ready-made salad dressings contain sugar. So too do fruits, sweetcorn and some other vegetables. As stated before, using the Carbs & Cals app is to me one of the best ways of working out the quantity of carbohydrate in your meal. Essentially you then add up all the carbohydrate on your plate or in your meal and convert that into an insulin dose.

Let's take the example of a packed lunch, containing a ham salad sandwich, using medium wholemeal bread, a medium apple and a packet of crisps or chips. The carbohydrates in each part of this are as follows:

Two slices of bread (15g each)	30g
Ham	nil
Salad	nil (well a few to be precise)
Apple	15g
Crisps/chips	13g
Total	58g

You could safely round this up to 60g, knowing that there likely to be one or two grams in the salad.

- If your ICR is 1 unit for 10g, then your insulin dose is 6 units: 60 x 1 ÷ 10 = 6.
- If your ICR is 1.5 units for 10g, then your insulin dose is 9 units: 60 x 1.5 ÷ 10 = 9.
- If your ICR is 1 unit per 8g, then your dose is 60 x 1 ÷ 8 = 7.5. You can round this down to 7 if your glucose level is normal or a little low, or round it up to 8 if your glucose level is a little high.

Let's try another example, of an evening meal of steak in a pepper sauce, peas, mushrooms and a small portion of mashed potato:

Steak	nil
Pepper sauce	5g
Peas	10g
Mushrooms	nil
Mashed potato	40g
Total	55g

- If your ICR is 1 unit for 10g, then your insulin dose is 5 or 6 units: 55 x 1 ÷ 10 = 5.5. You can round this down to 5 if your glucose level is normal or a little low, or round it up to 6 if your glucose level is a little high. Alternatively, you might have 6 units and a bit more potato!
- If your ICR is 1.5 units for 10g, then your insulin dose is 8 units: 55 x 1.5 ÷ 10 = 8.25. This can be safely rounded down to 8 units (or up to 9 with more potato).
- If your ICR is 1 unit per 8g, then your dose is 55 x 1 ÷ 8 = 6.9, which can be safely rounded up to 7 units.

I know that many people struggle with maths and for those that do, there are some glucose meters that do these calculations for you. They are termed automated bolus advisors, and will be discussed in more detail later in this chapter. These will be even more useful once we introduce correction doses that make the maths more complex.

CORRECTION DOSES – INTRODUCING THE INSULIN SENSITIVITY FACTOR

Sometimes, even when you have worked out the right ICR for you, you might underestimate the carbohydrate in a meal and inject too little insulin, or you might find your glucose level is high at lunchtime because you had a mid-morning snack. In the bad old days, people were told not to take extra insulin in such situations, which I know many found very frustrating. Nowadays, however, it is considered perfectly safe to take additional insulin to correct a high glucose level, as long as a number of important conditions are met. These are that:

1. Your basal insulin is doing a good job in keeping your glucose levels stable. This is particularly important when using correction doses at bedtime, as if the basal insulin brings the glucose level down overnight, there is an increased risk of a hypo during the night.

2. You do not give a correction dose if you had an injection of rapid-acting insulin within the previous three hours, as there will still be insulin on board. Or, if you do, that you know how to estimate the insulin on board and deduct it from the correction dose you are to give.

3. In view of this risk, as a rule you should add a correction dose to the next mealtime dose, or give as a bedtime dose, rather than

as an extra dose between meals. Exceptions to this rule would be if your glucose is already very high between meals and you are feeling unwell as a result, or if you are about to do some exercise.

4. You use an appropriate insulin sensitivity factor (ISF) to work out the correction dose and that you have an appropriate target level of glucose you are aiming to correct to. Both these are important to ensure that the correction dose you give is not too high, as this can lead to a really bad hypo.

The easier part of this is to set the target level. I generally suggest this to be set at 6mmol/l (110mg/dl), as it allows for a margin of error if the correction does work a bit too well. For example, if you set the target at 4mmol/l (70mg/dl) then there is no room for error as if the correction dose worked a bit too well you would have a hypo. I would generally suggest a slightly higher target level at bedtime, such as 7 or 8mmol/l (120 or 140mg/dl). If your glucose levels are running quite high, and especially if you have had bad experiences of correction doses in the past, it is reasonable to set a target level of 8mmol/l (140mg/dl) throughout the day, bearing in mind that this can always be adjusted in the future. In any case, it is important that you decide what level you are comfortable with setting as your initial target level.

Then to the ISF (insulin sensitivity factor). Essentially, this is an estimate of how much one unit of insulin will bring down the blood glucose level. In truth, it is very difficult to measure this accurately, and so it is important to err on the side of caution, to minimise any risk of hypoglycaemia. A usual starting ISF is for one unit of insulin to reduce the glucose level by 3mmol/l (or 50mg/dl), with a more gentle ISF at bedtime, initially at least 4mmol/l (or 70mg/dl). However, if you have low insulin requirements, such as a total of 30 units a day or less, or if your ICR is less than 1 unit per 10g of carbohydrate, then I would suggest an ISF of 4mmol/l (70mg/dl) during the day and 5mmol/l (90mg/dl) at bedtime.

Now we have to convert this into a correction dose. To do this, you need to check your blood glucose, then take away the target glucose level, and divide the result by the ISF.

Due to the complexity, the calculation steps are shown separately for those using mmol/l and mg/dl. Please note that, for this illustration, the example glucose levels are not exactly equivalent.

In mmol/l

So, if your glucose is 18mmol/l, you need to subtract the target glucose (6mmol/l) to get 18 – 6 = 12. Then you divide by your ISF (12 ÷ 3) to get 4 units. This is then added to the mealtime dose you are about to take.

If your glucose level was 17mmol/l, the correction dose would come out as 17 – 6 = 11, divided by 3 = 3.7. On the basis that it is always best to err on the side of caution, I would round this down to 3 units, initially at least. With experience, you may feel confident in rounding up (in this case to 4 units).

If your glucose level at bedtime was 18, you would use the bedtime ISF of 4. So, the calculation is 18 – 6 = 12, divided by 4 = 3, so the correction dose is 3 units to be taken at bedtime.

As a rule, you would not use a correction dose unless your glucose level is higher than your target BG + your ISF, i.e. 6 + 3 = 9 mmol/L or 6 + 4 = 10mmol/l at bedtime.

You can also use a negative correction dose if your glucose level is too low. For example, if your ICR is 1 unit for 10 grams and your ISF is one unit to reduce your glucose by 3mmol/l, you are about to eat a meal with 30 grams of carbohydrate and your glucose is 3.9mmol/l, then you can adjust the dose as follows:

Your usual dose would be 30 ÷ 10 = 3. However, as your glucose is below your target of 6 and is too low, you can reduce the dose by one unit, to allow the level to rise by 3mmol/l (your ISF), so you would take 2 units. The maths for this is as follows:

As the correction dose is calculated by subtracting your target glucose from your current glucose and dividing by your ISF, this would be $3.9 - 6 = -2.1$, divided by your ICR, which is 3, to give a correction dose of -0.7 units, that is you give 0.7 units less than you otherwise would. Unless you use a pump, then you can safely round this up to -1 unit, that is you take one unit off from your mealtime dose, to give $3 - 1 = 2$ units.

In reality, you should never need to reduce by more than one unit for a negative correction dose and can therefore save yourself the trouble of doing the calculation, and just reduce your dose by one unit if your glucose level is below your target level before you eat.

In mg/dl

If your BG is 310mg/dl, you need to subtract the target glucose (110mmol/l) to get $310 - 110 = 200$. Then you divide by your ISF (50) to get $200 \div 50 = 4$ units. This is then added to the mealtime dose you are about to take.

If your glucose level was 295, the correction dose would come out as $295 - 110 = 185$, divided by $50 = 3.7$. On the basis that it is always best to err on the side of caution, I would round this down to 3 units, initially at least. With experience, you may feel confident in rounding up (in this case to 4 units).

If your glucose level at bedtime was 310, you would use the bedtime ISF of 70. So the calculation is $310 - 70 = 240$, divided by $70 = 3.4$ so the correction dose is 3 units to be taken at bedtime.

As a rule, you would not use a correction dose unless your glucose level is higher than your target BG + your ISF, i.e. $110 + 50 = 160$mg/dl or $110 + 70 = 180$mg/dl at bedtime.

You can also use a negative correction dose if your glucose level is too low. For example, if your ICR is 1 unit for 10 grams and your ISF is one unit to reduce your glucose by 50mg/dl, you are about to eat a meal with 30 grams of carbohydrate and your glucose is 70mg/dl, then you can adjust the dose as follows:

Your usual dose would be 30 ÷ 10 = 3. However, as your glucose is below your target of 105 and is too low, you can reduce the dose by one unit, to allow the level to rise by 50mg/dl (your ISF), so you would take 2 units.

The calculation for this is as follows:

As the correction dose is calculated by subtracting your target glucose from your current glucose and dividing by your ISF, this would be 70 – 105 = -35, divided by your ICR, which is 50, to give a correction dose of -0.7 units. That is, you would give 0.7 units less than you otherwise would. Unless you use a pump, then you can safely round this up to -1 unit, so take one unit off from your mealtime dose, to give 3 – 1 = 2 units.

In reality, you should never need to reduce by more than one unit for a negative correction dose and can therefore save yourself the trouble of doing the calculation, and just reduce your dose by one unit if your glucose level is below your target level before you eat.

For the mathematically-minded, the equation used to work out your bolus dose, i.e. your meal dose plus correction dose is:

((Current BG level – target BG level) ÷ ISF) + (ICR x grams carbohydrate ÷ 10) if you use an ICR expressed as the number of units for each 10 grams of carbohydrate, or

((Current BG level – target BG level) ÷ ISF) + (grams carbohydrate ÷ ICR) if you use an ICR expressed as the number of grams for each unit of insulin.

From this, an estimate of 'insulin on board' should be subtracted if applicable.

A colleague of mine once asked a university mathematics lecturer about this calculation. They acknowledged that it was a very complex calculation. However, please do not let this put you off beginning to use the ICR and ISF. With time, you will find that you automatically know the amount of carbohydrate in your favourite foods, and how to work out a correction dose when necessary. Once you know your ISF, you can easily write out a chart such as these below to help you with corrections:

Using mmol/L

My ISF is 3mmol/l. That means that 1 unit of insulin will reduce my blood glucose by 3mmol/l. My target BG is 6mmol/l.

At bedtime, my ISF is 4mmol/l and my target BG is 8mmol/l.

Daytime – to add to meal dose			Bedtime	
Glucose level	Correction dose		Glucose level	Correction dose
Less than 6	-1 units		Less than 8	Eat 10g carbohydrate*
Less than 9	0 units		Less than 12	0 units
9–11.9	1 units		12–15.9	1 units
12–14.9	2 units		16–19.9	2 units
15–17.9	3 units		20–23	3 units
18–20.9	4 units			
21–23	5 units			

*As you would not normally give a bolus at bedtime, you cannot use a negative correction dose. In this situation, you could eat 10 grams of carbohydrate. Another option, if you also give your basal insulin at bedtime, would be to reduce this by 1–2 units, although this may then affect your glucose control the next day.

Using mg/dl

My ISF is 50mg/dl. That means that 1 unit of insulin will reduce my blood glucose by 50mg/dl. My target BG is 110mg/dl.

At bedtime, my ISF is 70mg/dl and my target BG is 140mg/dl.

Daytime – to add to meal dose			Bedtime	
Glucose level	**Correction dose**		**Glucose level**	**Correction dose**
Less than 110	-1 unit		Less than 140	Eat 10g carbohydrate*
Less than 160	0 units		Less than 210	0 units
160–210	1 units		210–280	1 units
211–260	2 units		281–350	2 units
261–310	3 units		351–420	3 units
311–360	4 units			
361–410	5 units			

*As you would not normally give a bolus at bedtime, you cannot use a negative correction dose. In this situation, you could eat 10 grams of carbohydrate. Another option, if you also give your basal insulin at bedtime, would be to reduce this by 1–2 units, although this may then affect your glucose control the next day.

Once you have given a correction dose, it is important to remember that it can take up to three hours before the glucose reaches your target level. While you may wish to check it an hour later, it is not advisable to take any additional insulin unless the glucose level is still too high at least three hours later (or before your next meal). If you do, you are at high risk of having a hypo.

In the previous chapter, we discussed how, in some people, an injection of basal insulin might run out at certain times of the day, allowing the glucose to rise. If this occurs with you, and it is not possible or appropriate to switch to a different basal insulin, or use a pump, then this can be addressed by using a correction dose, calculated as described above and added to your mealtime dose(s).

MEALS WITH VERY FEW CARBOHYDRATES

Let's look at a variation of the steak meal mentioned earlier, that consists of steak with herb butter, spinach, mushrooms and 'cauliflower mash'.

Steak	nil
Herb butter	nil
Spinach	1g
Mushrooms	2g
Cauliflower mash	5g
Total	8g

In this case, you can see that you will need at most 1 unit of insulin, and quite possibly none at all. This is a good example of how choosing a meal with low-carbohydrate ingredients significantly reduces, or eliminates, the need for mealtime insulin. You might choose to do this if you are eating out, or if for any other reason you do not want the hassle of having to inject insulin. For example, you might be out and about and expect to do a lot of walking, and would prefer to have less insulin on board to reduce the risk of having a hypo. Whatever the reason, it is perfectly acceptable to choose a very low-carbohydrate meal, and some people choose this for all their meals, as will be discussed in more detail in chapter 12. I would still recommend that you check your blood glucose beforehand, in case you need to give a correction dose, but some people will choose not to do this, and wait until they get home to check their glucose level.

Many of my patients have found that they get the best control of their glucose levels when they have low carbohydrate meals, and as a result my general recommendation is to try and keep the carbs in any one meal to 30 grams or less. As with all my recommendations, these are just that – suggestions for day-to-day living. However, they can of course be over-ruled for a special occasion or a meal out.

LARGE CARBOHYDRATE MEALS

Ten years ago, I believed that if you used modern insulin analogues, knew how to count your carbohydrates and adjust your insulin, then you could eat whatever you liked. With a decade more experience, wisdom and also common sense, I firmly believe that is not the case. Thus, I no longer say you can have a large deep pan pizza and keep your blood glucose under control. However, if that is a meal you enjoy from time to time, there are certain tips that can help ensure your glucose levels avoid roller-coaster highs and lows.

A 12" deep pan pizza can have anything up to 200 grams of carbohydrate. Now, regardless of your ICR, this will add up to a very large dose. If you took it all at once, there is a risk that the insulin would kick in before you have had much of the pizza and put you at risk of a hypo. This is particularly an issue for meals that combine a lot of fat with carbohydrate, as the fat (in this case in the cheese in the pizza) tends to delay the absorption of the carbohydrate and so slows down the rate at which glucose appears in the bloodstream. There is also a risk that you get halfway through the pizza and just cannot eat any more – yet you have had enough insulin for all of it. So, either you must finish it or risk having a hypo.

This is a situation where a split bolus would be advised, that means, having some insulin at the start of the meal and some at the end. If you calculate that the total insulin required for the pizza is 20 units, then I would suggest giving between a third to a half before you start eating, and the remainder at the end. Having a later second dose will prolong the overall effect of the dose, to take into account the slow absorption because of all the fat in the meal. It will also enable you to give the amount you need for the total carbohydrate you actually ate, rather than what you thought you would eat, and thus avoid the risk of a hypo.

So, if the dose for the whole pizza is 20 units, in this example you would give, say 8 units at the start, and then the rest at the end. If you ate all the pizza, that would be an additional 12 units. However, if you only manage to eat three-quarters of the pizza, then the total dose required would be ¾ of 20, which equals 15 units. As you have already given 8, then you need to give another 7 at the end. This same principle would apply for all large carbohydrate meals such as pasta dishes (lasagne, macaroni cheese, spaghetti Bolognese), rice dishes and potato dishes. Note though that white rice and potato are more quickly absorbed than pasta or pizza (unless there is also a lot of fat in the meal).

There is another good reason to consider avoiding a single large dose of insulin, and that is that there is a tendency for a large dose to be absorbed more slowly than a smaller dose. This is a result of the physical property of a small dose that means it will be absorbed into your system much quicker than a large dose. For those who are interested in physics, it has to do with the fact that a small 'bubble' of insulin that has been injected has a large surface area compared to its volume, and so the insulin in the middle of the 'bubble' will quickly get to the surface and be rapidly absorbed. A large dose, on the other hand creates a large 'bubble' with a relatively small surface area compared to its volume, and so the insulin in the middle of the large 'bubble' can take some time until it gets to the surface and is absorbed.

For this reason, some people make it a rule never to inject more than six units of fast-acting insulin in one injection. If they need to inject twelve units, they would inject two doses of six units at the same time, but into different sites. Obviously, if you are using an insulin pump this is not possible, but most pumps allow for split or prolonged (so-called 'square wave' or 'multiwave') boluses that will have the same effect, and these will be covered in more detail in chapter 13.

EATING OUT

Eating out is another situation where a split dose is not only a good option, but often essential. We all enjoy going to a restaurant and eating a meal of two, three or even more courses. Very few of us know exactly what we will eat, and how much of it, and when, right at the start. Yes, you may have chosen your starter and main course, but until it arrives you don't know how much carbohydrate there will be on the plate, nor how much of it you will eat. Many of us have also had the experience of waiting a very long time for food to arrive, and if you have given a large dose of insulin with no food appearing for forty minutes, you will be at high risk of a hypo. I recall many years ago, in the time when many people took a large fixed dose of insulin before their evening meal, being in a restaurant where at another table there was a young lady who did just that. As time went by she became more and more anxious, and before long was tucking into a bowlful of sugar as she began to feel very hypo.

The ideal solution to a meal out would be to have an insulin dose for each course as it arrives and after you have estimated the carbohydrate content and how much of it you might eat. If you are not sure you will eat all the carbohydrate, then you can inject half and top up later, perhaps adding it to the 'dessert' dose. Note that generally, you only need to check your blood glucose before the first injection, in case you need to include a correction dose.

If you have an insulin pump, then it is easy to give several boluses. However, if you inject each dose with a syringe or insulin pen you may wish to avoid multiple injections, although in most cases two will be necessary unless you opt for carbohydrate-free choices. This can be done as follows:

1. Aim to have a starter with no or very little carbohydrate, such as a salad or garlic mushrooms (without breadcrumbs).
2. Inject the first bolus as you start the main course, to cover any carbohydrate in the starter plus what you think you will eat in the main course.
3. Inject the second bolus to cover any top-up for the main course plus any dose needed for dessert. This can be given either before you start the dessert or immediately after you finish. The advantage of the latter is that you will know exactly how much you have eaten and can take into account any extra, such as helping someone else finish theirs!

ADJUSTING BOLUS DOSES FOR THE EFFECTS OF PROTEIN AND FAT

The body does not actually need any carbohydrate from our food, as it can make glucose from other food sources according to need, including from protein. Thus, some protein is converted into glucose. I have met some diabetes specialists who routinely advise their patients to take some insulin for protein as well as carbohydrate. A recent review has suggested that the glucose rise from protein occurs about two hours after the meal[27] and can cause glucose levels to be raised for up to 5 hours after the meal.[28] Having a meal with protein only (and no fat or carbohydrate) appeared to have little effect on blood glucose values unless over 75 grams of protein was consumed. This amount of protein had a similar effect on the blood glucose level as 20 grams of carbohydrate, suggesting it might be appropriate to have a small dose of insulin after the meal.[29]

Fat in a meal can also affect the amount of insulin needed. The body converts fat to fatty acids that reduce the effect of insulin on the liver, leading to higher glucose levels and so in theory this increases the amount of insulin required. One study suggested that 50 grams of fat in a meal required one person to need a double dose of insulin.[30] However, it is also the case that fat delays the absorption of carbohydrate and thus there is an increased risk of hypoglycaemia if all the bolus is given before the meal. Thus, if you have a meal with a high fat content, it would be worth considering splitting the dose and having part of the dose after the meal (or having an extended bolus if you are using an insulin pump, see chapter 13).

One method of working out how to correct for protein or fat is the Warsaw formula[31] that suggests one unit of insulin is added for every 100 calories in a meal derived from protein or fat. Another is to use the Food Insulin Index (FII) to calculate the insulin required for individual foods.[32] These are primarily designed for insulin pump users as it is suggested doses are given as an extended bolus over a few hours. It also requires a level of complexity to know how to estimate the calorie as well as carbohydrate content of meals, and I for one would struggle with that.

Counting carbohydrates and calculating insulin doses is complicated enough, without adding in the complexities that fat and protein also bring. Therefore, I suggest that you base your insulin doses on carbohydrate alone in the first instance, and then make adjustments based on your experience of high fat or high protein meals. A pragmatic approach, that I recommend, is to correct for any lasting effect of a high-protein or high-fat meal by applying a correction dose to the next mealtime dose, or as a bedtime correction dose in the evening.

AUTOMATED BOLUS ADVISORS

By now you will have gathered that calculating the amount of insulin required for your mealtime dose is complex. You may be forgiven for thinking that it is much easier just to take the same dose with every meal. That is an option, but unless you are diligent in ensuring that you eat the same amount of carbohydrate at the same time every day, and do the same amount of physical activity, then this will likely lead to widely fluctuating glucose levels. Another option is to use an automated bolus advisor, a type of calculator that is built into a blood glucose meter. There are two such meters currently available, the Accu-chek Aviva Expert meter, manufactured by Roche, and the Freestyle Insulinx, made by Abbott.

With both products, when you perform a blood glucose measurement, the meters suggest an insulin dose for you to take. In order for them to do this, the meters have to be set up with your personal settings for ICR and ISF, and also your target glucose value. These can vary for different times of the day. When you want the meter to calculate an insulin dose, as well as measuring your blood glucose, you then need to enter the amount of carbohydrate you intend to eat. Note that the Insulinx does have the option of an easy mode, for people who use fixed insulin doses for meals, for which it is not necessary to enter the carbohydrate content; using this option, the meter simply suggests a correction dose, if required. This is not ideal for people with type 1 diabetes and I will not discuss it further here. There are other important differences in the meters, as described in the table below.

Feature	Expert meter	Insulinx meter
Customised to individual's parameters: ICR, ISF and target blood glucose value:	Yes – and the user can adjust parameters as required	Yes – but only a health professional can set and adjust these (password-protected)
Ability to have different ICR, ISF and target glucose values at different times of day:	Yes – each can be set for any number of different 'time blocks' through the 24-hour period.	Yes – but the 'time blocks' are fixed: 6 to 10am, 10am to 4pm, 4pm to 10pm, 10pm to 6am
Ability to set the duration of insulin action:	Yes	Yes – in advanced mode only
Ability to adjust the dose for exercise, stress or illness:	Yes	No
Ability to keep track of previously injected 'insulin on board':	Yes – insulin on board is known as 'active insulin'.	Yes – but will not suggest correction dose if any insulin has been injected within the past two hours
Ability to download and view blood glucose data:	Yes – in interactive format that enables data to be viewed in different ways	Yes – in a standard static form

You will see that the Expert meter allows for a greater number of different settings during the day, and takes into account lifestyle factors such as stress and illness (for which the meter can be set to increase the suggested dose by a certain percentage) and exercise (for which the meter can be set to decrease the dose). The data from the Expert meter can also be downloaded and viewed interactively at your diabetes clinic, or indeed at home, whereas the Insulinx provides static reports that are not interactive.

The greatest advantage of the Expert meter is that the settings can be adjusted by the user, and I encourage users to do this, once they feel confident in doing so. The Insulinx, on the other hand, may be more suitable for people who do not feel confident in changing their insulin to carbohydrate ratio or other settings.

With both meters, once they have been set up with your settings, as long as you tell the meter how much carbohydrate you will eat once you have done the blood test, it will do all the calculations for you and provide a suggested insulin dose, without the need for any mental arithmetic on your part. Such bolus advisors can therefore be very helpful, especially with the complex calculations that are required to determine mealtime insulin doses. However, they are only as good as the data that have been entered, including the ICR and ISF, and so it is very important that you take some time to determine the correct ICR(s) and ISF(s) for you, and that you have a full understanding of how the doses are calculated and why, before relying on an automated advisor for your doses. It is also important to realise that the meters only advise on mealtime or correction doses, not on the basal insulin dose. Indeed, they assume that the basal insulin dose has been set correctly, and keeps the glucose level stable, as discussed in chapter 10. It is therefore very important that you have been through these steps to optimise your basal insulin, before using one of these meters.

A number of studies have been carried out to test the benefit of these meters. The most extensive was ABACUS, the Automated Bolus Advisor Control and Usability Study,[33] that evaluated the Expert meter. This showed that a greater number of users of the Expert meter were able to improve their HbA1c by more than 0.5 per cent (or 6mmol/mol) than those who used a standard glucose meter. The Expert users also improved their accuracy in carbohydrate counting and reported better satisfaction with their treatment. This was also borne out in the many patients who used the Expert meter while I was working at the Bournemouth Diabetes Clinic. Now in truth, not everyone used the meter to calculate every insulin dose, but many of those that did found it invaluable, and many saw their diabetes control improve. A number of reports have also demonstrated benefits of using the

Insulinx, although these were mainly in people using it in 'easy mode'.[34,35]

On the basis of my own clinical experience, and the greater functionality, I do prefer the Expert meter for people with type 1 diabetes who estimate their insulin doses using carbohydrate counting. However, it is important that I state here that I was one of the investigators that helped design the ABACUS study, and so perhaps I am biased in favour of the Expert meter. Therefore, if you are considering one of these meters, you may wish to discuss their pros and cons with a diabetes specialist nurse or educator.

I am aware that this has been quite a complex chapter, but that emphasises the challenge of getting the right insulin dose for each meal you eat. If you are new to these methods of calculating your mealtime insulin, and you find them confusing, I would suggest you seek the advice of a specialist diabetes health professional who can help you. There is also lots of support available via Internet forums. Above all, I would urge you to persevere with the new learning as, in the long term, I am convinced that it offers a much better way of achieving stable blood glucose values than using fixed insulin doses. Furthermore, over time, you will quickly learn how much insulin you need to give for each of your favourite meals, and the calculations that now may seem very complex, will begin to become less onerous.

12

A HEALTHY DIET FOR TYPE 1 DIABETES

The standard dietary advice for everyone, issued by Public Health England, is to base meals on the Eatwell Guide. This shows the proportions of the main food groups that form a healthy, balanced diet.

The recommendations can be summarised as follows:

▶ Eat at least 5 portions of a variety of fruit and vegetables every day;

▶ Base meals on potatoes, bread, rice, pasta or other starchy carbohydrates – choosing wholegrain versions where possible;

▶ Have some dairy or dairy alternatives (such as soya drinks), choosing lower fat and lower sugar options;

▶ Eat some beans, pulses, fish, eggs, meat and other proteins (including 2 portions of fish every week, one of which should be oily);

- Choose unsaturated oils and spreads and eat in small amounts;
- Drink 6–8 cups/glasses of fluid a day;
- If consuming foods and drinks high in fat, salt or sugar, have these less often and in small amounts.

Until relatively recently, the standard advice for people with type 1 diabetes was to follow the same diet as that recommended for the general population, namely to base all meals on starchy carbohydrates and to limit fat intake. As I discussed earlier, there was a time when it was felt as long as you took the right dose of insulin, then you could essentially eat as much carbohydrate as you like. In the past ten years, however, an increasing number of people working in diabetes, as well as people with type 1 diabetes themselves, have come to realise that this advice doesn't seem entirely logical for a person whose metabolism, by definition, cannot handle carbohydrates. I am one of those who firmly believes that the standard advice is not likely to enable people with type 1 diabetes to achieve stable blood glucose control.

LOW CARB, HEALTHY FAT (LCHF)

The Public Health Collaboration is an independent group of health professionals with an interest and expertise in nutritional matters. They believe that a high carbohydrate diet is positively harmful for the general population, for whom they have produced their own version of the Eatwell guide, as shown below. Note that the emphasis is on eating real, unprocessed foods, restricting carbohydrates to less than 130 grams a day and using healthy fats such as are found in dairy products, nuts, olives, avocadoes and good quality meat.

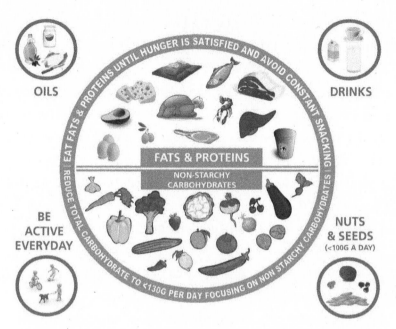

Reproduced by kind permission of the Public Health Collaboration[36]

Note also that this is very different from the Eatwell Guide. Gone is the large portion recommending starchy carbohydrates. Gone also is the recommendation to use low fat products, that by definition are processed and unnatural and often come with added sugar. Instead, adopting the PHC diet will mean avoiding most processed foods, eating large quantities of fresh vegetables and some low-sugar fruits, and excluding foods with added sugars completely.

Even if the Eatwell Guide is a good idea for the general population, the official advice that people with diabetes should base their meals on carbohydrates does seem rather bizarre. A person with type 1 diabetes cannot handle carbohydrates properly; it is a form of carbohydrate intolerance. In almost any other type of food intolerance, the advice would be to restrict or eliminate those foods to which you are intolerant. And this was the basis of the standard 'diabetic diet' right up to the 1970s. I recently met a lady who worked as a nurse with Dr RD Lawrence and who lent me a treasured copy of the final edition of his book, *The Diabetic ABC: A Practical Guide for Patients and Nurses*, published in 1964. He had type 1 diabetes and was one of the first people in the UK to receive insulin in the 1923. He then went on to become a specialist in diabetes and in his book he described his recommended diet for people with diabetes.[37] The basic recommendation was to restrict carbohydrates to about 100 grams per day, which could be increased to 150g to include snacks necessary to prevent hypoglycaemia due to the insulins used at the time. He followed such a diet and lived to the age of 76 after a long and illustrious career and 45 years of living with diabetes, quite remarkable in those days.

Over the past 20 years, despite the advances in insulin treatments, in pump technology and in monitoring techniques, many people with type 1 diabetes still struggle to achieve stable control. That led me to question the current advice that promotes a high carbohydrate intake, and for the past several years I have recommended carbohydrate restriction, just as Dr Lawrence did. So, what are the benefits of carbohydrate restriction? The most obvious one is that if you are eating less carbohydrate, then your food will have less effect in raising your blood glucose levels. That in turn will mean you need to inject less insulin. Less insulin means less chance of having a hypo, and more chance of stable blood glucose levels. Less insulin also means that the amount of insulin in your circulation will be less, and so there is less risk of the consequences of too much insulin. One of these is hunger, and many people who are on too much insulin report that they always feel hungry. This of course contributes to another result of too much insulin, that is weight gain, which I have seen very often in people who have been on high doses of insulin. With weight gain come other associated problems, and one of these is insulin resistance. This describes the situation where the body is unable to use insulin effectively, and that the insulin has less effect in reducing blood glucose levels. If this happens, you may find you need to increase your ICR and ISF and possibly also your basal insulin dose. So you end up with even more circulating insulin that leads to more weight gain and more insulin resistance, creating a vicious cycle. This is seen in many people with type 2 diabetes. In recent years, many with type 2 diabetes have found that carbohydrate restriction enables them to achieve better blood glucose levels, to lose weight, and in some cases to reverse their diabetes completely. Now, type 1 diabetes is of course very different, but my experience of treating people with type 2 diabetes with carbohydrate restriction has convinced me of the benefits also in people with type 1 diabetes, especially those who are overweight or who are on large doses of insulin.

A number of studies have looked at the evidence to support carbohydrate restriction in type 1 diabetes. In a study from Sweden, 48 people with type 1 diabetes adopted a low-carbohydrate diet (between 70 and 90 grams a day) and were followed up for four years. Their average HbA1c fell from 7.6 to 6.9 per cent (58 to 52 mmol/mol). Those that followed the low-carbohydrate diet most reliably did best, with an average HbA1c of 6 per cent (42 mmol/mol) at four years, and their mealtime insulin dose nearly halved from 21 to 12 units a day. What was really striking was that during the first year, episodes of hypoglycaemia fell dramatically from nearly 3 a week on average to one every two weeks. Some individuals saw dramatic improvements in their blood glucose control; in one person, their average blood glucose on their usual diet was 12.9mmol/l (232mg/dl) and this fell to 5.9mmol/l (106mg/dl) on the low carbohydrate diet, with much less variation in values.[38]

Another study, this time from New Zealand, showed the benefit of a low-carbohydrate diet.[39] It looked at ten people with longstanding type 1 diabetes, who on average had a body mass index of 27, indicating that they were overweight. Five went on to a low-carbohydrate diet for 12 weeks, aiming for 75 grams a day. The others stayed on their usual diet. After 12 weeks, the low-carbohydrate group reduced their insulin dose by a third (from 64 to 44 units a day), lost an average of 5kg (11lb) in weight and saw a reduction in their HbA1c from 7.9 to 7.2 per cent (63 to 55mmol/mol). The other group saw no such changes. The low-carbohydrate group reduced their carbohydrate intake from an average of 219g to 103g per day, somewhat higher than the 75g advised. Interestingly, they did not increase their fat intake and their total calories each day reduced from 1988 to 1391. They were overweight and so did not need to take extra fat to make up for the energy lost from reducing carbohydrate. Interestingly, some found that they needed more insulin than they would have expected for some meals and this suggests that some of the protein eaten could have been converted into glucose (as explained in chapter 11).

Some people assume that a low carbohydrate diet has to be high in fat, hence the term 'low carb, high fat' or LCHF diet. However this study shows that this doesn't have to be the case. In someone who is not overweight, increasing the portion of protein or of healthy fats, as recommended by the PHC, can make up for the reduced carbohydrates. Thus I prefer to use the term 'Low Carb, *Healthy Fat*' to describe the diet, as by avoiding processed foods that contain harmful trans-fats, and by eating fat found naturally in foods, that is just what it is.

The above studies would suggest that there is good evidence that an intake of 70–100 grams of carbohydrate is an effective and sustainable means of improving glucose control in people with diabetes. This ties in with my own recommendation, and interestingly is similar to those of Dr Lawrence. However, I would encourage you to find the level that works well for you and fits in with your own tastes and food preferences. As with all my recommendations, this is what is recommended for day-to-day living. You can of course allow yourself exceptions, when eating out or on special occasions, and using your ICR will allow you to give the right amount of insulin for larger carbohydrate meals.

KETOGENIC DIET AND TYPE 1 DIABETES

A ketogenic diet is a true Low Carbohydrate High Fat Diet. This is a diet where the carbohydrate intake is restricted to less than 50 grams a day, and protein is also restricted so that the body predominantly burns fat for energy, a process called ketosis.

A ketogenic diet can be used to help people lose weight, predominantly body fat, and it is one means of promoting reversal of type 2 diabetes. It has recently also come to light as an option for people with type 1 diabetes. Before discussing this further, it is important to distinguish ketosis, which occurs in people who follow a ketogenic diet, from ketoacidosis, the condition that arises in people with type 1 diabetes when they have insufficient insulin. In both conditions, the ketone level in the blood or urine will be raised as a result of the body predominantly burning fat for energy. The key difference of course is that nutritional ketosis results from an intentional diet that is low in carbohydrate, while insulin injections are maintained and blood glucose levels are kept under control. Ketoacidosis, on the other hand, as described in chapter 4, results from lack of insulin, leading to high levels of glucose in the bloodstream. As the tissues cannot access this glucose for energy, fat is used instead, resulting in high ketone levels.

A ketogenic diet means that carbohydrate is not required and thus very little or no mealtime insulin is required, apart from correction doses or insulin needed for protein or fat. One of the earliest advocates of a very low-carbohydrate diet for type 1 diabetes was Dr Richard Bernstein. Dr Bernstein developed type 1 diabetes in 1946 at the age of 12, and after twenty years was beginning to experience many of the problems associated with longstanding type 1 diabetes. In the late 1960s, he purchased one of the very first blood glucose analysers and for the first time – and years before most other people with diabetes – began to measure his own glucose levels. This led him on a journey to his developing and adopting a very low-carbohydrate diet to enable him to manage his diabetes with HbA1c levels around 4 per cent (20mmol/mol). He was originally an engineer, and used his analytical skills to develop a different way to manage his own diabetes. He describes his approach in his book published in 1997, *Dr Bernstein's Diabetes Solution*.[40] His approach is quite restrictive in terms of what can and cannot be eaten. The maximum carbohydrate that he allows is 30 grams per day (6 with breakfast, 12 each with lunch and the evening meal) and that precludes all fruits except avocadoes and many vegetables. Alongside the dietary restriction, he developed detailed methods to calculate the effect of insulin in reducing blood glucose levels and to determine the amount of insulin needed, with the precision that you would expect from an engineer. He worked on the basis that avoiding carbohydrates means that there is one less factor at work (that is, diet) in affecting blood glucose levels. His goal was to keep his glucose levels as normal and as stable as possible, and using what we would now call 'old-fashioned' insulins, he got impressive results. Not only did his glucose control improve, so too did his health. Many of the problems that resulted from his diabetes began to resolve. In his book, he writes: *'After years of chronic fatigue and debilitating complications, almost overnight I was no longer continually tired or "washed out" … I started to gain weight, and at last I was able to build muscle as readily as non-diabetics.'* He goes on to relate how his insulin requirements dropped to one-fifth of what they were previously and how his digestive problems and the protein in his urine cleared up. So determined was he to get this message out there, and equally frustrated that as a non-doctor his voice was not heard, that he changed career and at the age of 45 trained as a doctor so that he could set up a medical practice in which he would go on to share his approach with people with both type 1 and type 2 diabetes with great success.

Although he does not expressly mention ketosis as part of his regimen, such restriction of carbohydrate intake will normally be associated with ketosis, or using fat as the main source of energy. One person who has adopted this approach more recently is Dr Ian Lake, a medical doctor who describes his experiences in a blog at Type1keto.com.[41] He tells how he developed a late-onset form of type 1 diabetes at the age of 35. For nearly twenty years he followed the standard advice to have a low fat, high carbohydrate diet. He regarded himself as a healthy and active person. He attended all his clinic visits and did his best to follow the rules, but his fluctuating blood glucose levels began to take their toll. On his blog, he writes '*You see, I was getting desperate. I had had a few hypo crises, slightly more unannounced than before. Not unmanageable but I was needing to be more careful. They were a brooding shadow over my outdoor active lifestyle. And, worse, I was feeling old, with joint aches, general stiffness and generally fogged thought. Nothing specific, just below what I felt should be normal. I was also injecting higher doses of insulin with no improvement in control. Not a good place to be.*'

He accepted this was part and parcel of living with type 1 diabetes and that the diabetes was now beginning to take its toll. Then he read Dr Bernstein's book and was inspired to try and improve his health. In 2015, he adopted a ketogenic diet containing about 30 grams of carbohydrate per day. He reports that he found it difficult to reject the previous advice on fats and carbohydrates that he had believed in for the previous twenty years of having diabetes. His new diet contained 30–50 grams of carbohydrate and at first up to half of this was in the form of sugar to help stabilise his glucose levels and avoid hypoglycaemia. Very quickly his insulin requirements reduced significantly and, with smaller doses of insulin, his blood glucose levels were smoothed out. Hypos became much rarer and easier to manage. Following the change to his diet, he wrote, '*I now feel good. Vital in fact, with a marked improvement in clarity of thinking and vision, gradually reducing weight, absence of joint pains and improved stamina. My HbA1c has improved and I am aiming to get into the normal range in the next year. I now actually look forward to getting tested rather than hoping that I am still getting away with it.*'

As stated, I generally advise to limit carbohydrate to no more than 30 grams at any one meal, and to aim for 75 to 100 grams per day, as this reduces insulin requirements and variability in blood glucose levels. However, Dr Bernstein has shown that a much lower carbohydrate intake is also possible and may be preferable in some people. I do not have enough experience of working with people with type 1 diabetes on very-low-carbohydrate diets to make a specific recommendation, however I would not dissuade anyone who wanted to try such an approach for themselves. After all, humans do not actually need any carbohydrate in their diet.

Having said that, if you do aim for a very-low-carbohydrate diet, your body may take some time to get used to it. As it does so, you may experience some temporary side effects, sometimes called 'carb flu'. The most common symptoms include lethargy, leg cramps, constipation and palpitations. These are due to the body acclimatising to having less available glucose from carbohydrates and having to use fat for energy instead. Once the body does acclimatise, then these symptoms resolve, usually after a few days. They can be minimised by making sure you drink sufficient water, and ensuring there is enough salt in your diet. This is because one of the actions of insulin is to retain salt in the body; as you will now be having much less insulin, there is a risk you will become somewhat deficient in salt. It is suggested therefore that you add a total 5 grams of salt (about a teaspoon) each day to your meals. This can be split between 2 or 3 meals. For the same reason, if you have been taking medications for high blood pressure, these may need to be reduced as your blood pressure may fall quite steeply as, with less insulin on board, your body no longer retains so much water.

There is also a phenomenon in which in some people, adopting a ketotic diet can lead to high blood cholesterol levels. This is usually seen in healthy, lean people who have been described as 'lean-mass hyper-responders'.[42] It is likely that the high cholesterol levels reflect the fact that increased fat is being transported in the blood stream, rather than any underlying disease.

As with all things, there is no one solution that suits everyone. Some people choose to adopt a very low carbohydrate diet and live in a state of permanent ketosis; others (me included) would find the dietary restrictions that imposes too rigid, and opt for a higher carbohydrate intake. The important thing is that you find what works best for you.

13

INSULIN PUMP THERAPY

An insulin pump is a wearable device that releases an infusion of insulin into the subcutaneous tissue, usually through a fine tube or cannula. It contains a refillable reservoir which holds between 180 and 300 units of rapid-acting insulin (or soluble/regular insulin if rapid-acting insulin is not available). The pump delivers this as a continuous infusion to provide basal insulin. The basal rate can be tailored to each individual, and can vary throughout the 24-hour period. Most pumps allow for a number of different basal rates to cater for different situations, such as work days, non-work days or days when physical activity will be very different, for example for people who undertake regular exercise. The mealtime and correction boluses are delivered via the same route. These have to be set and delivered manually, by using the controls of the pump. Most of the time, bolus doses are calculated and given in the same way as with injected insulin, although insulin pumps do allow for different types of bolus for specific needs, as will be discussed later in this chapter. While the pump enables the user to give several boluses a day without needing to inject, and at much smaller doses than is possible with injections, the greatest advantage of using an insulin pump is its ability to deliver flexible basal rates.

The first insulin pumps were in use in the 1980s; however, in the UK at least, they tended to be reserved for people who had particular problems with managing their diabetes, in the mistaken belief that providing an insulin pump will sort those problems out. Not surprisingly, this didn't work. The pumps were also not as reliable as modern-day devices and some people experienced diabetic ketoacidosis as a result of the pump failing to deliver insulin. After a few years, they fell out of favour and pretty much disappeared from the diabetes landscape for many years.

The new pump era started in the late 1990s. In the US, and some European countries such as Germany, insulin pump use took off quite rapidly. Not so in the UK, where the combination of their high cost and lingering suspicion from the experience of the older generation of pumps, meant that their take-up was much slower. Indeed, I recall a meeting of the great and the good in the diabetes world in the year 2000, where I raised the importance of devoting more funding to insulin pumps. I was told in no uncertain terms that 'insulin pumps kill people'. Thankfully, I do not hear that sentiment nowadays. Many research studies have firmly established the benefits of using an insulin pump. Several have shown that using a pump is associated with better diabetes control with less risk of severe hypos, usually with lower insulin requirement.[43] Insulin pumps are therefore particularly useful for people who have experienced recurrent hypos on injections.

MY EXPERIENCE WITH INSULIN PUMP THERAPY

At the time I was working at the Diabetes Centre in Bournemouth, on the south coast of England. We were a forward-looking team and liked to bring in new ideas, and in 1998 Joan Everett, one of the nurse educators was despatched off to Germany and Switzerland to learn all about these new devices. Upon her return, the pump companies provided the department with some of their new models to test on willing patients, and the modern pump service was born. This was at about the same time as we were developing the early BERTIE education programmes and so at that time, carbohydrate counting was not widespread and the concepts of insulin-to-carbohydrate ratios and sensitivity factors were new to both patients and staff. Nevertheless, there was a belief that these concepts could be introduced quite rapidly and that the pump will be so good that patients were bound to benefit. Some did, and they did very well indeed. This was also before the time of the modern long-acting insulin analogues such as detemir or glargine, and so the only available basal insulins were the older isophane insulins. As we discussed in chapter 10, these were very variable in their effect and many people struggled with unpredictable hypoglycaemia, especially at night. They, especially, found almost immediate and great benefit from switching to an insulin pump. I well recall one lady in her thirties, who had struggled with her diabetes for many years, telling me in the outpatient clinic how she felt normal for the first time in her adult life. She described how she could go to bed without worrying about whether she would have a hypo; she said that the lack of hypos and more stable glucose levels resulted in her mood being more stable than she could ever remember – and her husband agreed! I was so struck by what she said that I asked my colleague (who had started her on the pump) to come in and hear what she had to say. It was one of those rare moments when you know that someone's life really has been revolutionised for the better.

Over the next few years, our team started 45 people on an insulin pump, and followed them up over two years. Over that time, their average HbA1c fell from 9.6 to 8.6 per cent (81 to 71mmol/mol) despite requiring on average a third less insulin (from 63 to 42 units) per day. They also lost an average of 2kg (4½lb) in weight and experienced a lot less hypoglycaemia – good news all round. At that time, insulin pumps were not yet available on the NHS and unless their pumps were provided as part of a clinical trial, people who wished to use a pump had to pay for it themselves. The cost was (and still is) prohibitive for most people, at £2–3,000 for the pump and at least another £1,000 for the consumables every year. Nevertheless, the early results encouraged us and others to press for better access to insulin pumps, and in 2003 the National Institute for Health and Clinical Excellence (NICE) provided its first guidance to enable pumps to be provided on the NHS. NICE stated that insulin pump therapy was an option for people with type 1 diabetes who are unable to achieve an HbA1c of 7.5 per cent (58mmol/mol) without disabling hypoglycaemia, who had commitment and competence, and if pump therapy is initiated by a trained specialist team comprising a physician, diabetic nurse specialist and dietitian. These very stringent rules were widely criticised, as there was an implication that in order to have access to a pump, you had to have had disabling hypoglycaemia; however, they did allow the slow start of what was to become a big expansion of the use of insulin pumps in the UK.

In the early years, pumps were only available at a few centres, with a 'trained specialist team'. Bournemouth was one of those and before long we were receiving referrals from a very wide area of patients who were felt to be in need of an insulin pump. At first we obliged, and put them on a pump; however it soon became apparent that many of these people were not actually doing much better on a pump than on injections. Many who had bad hypos on injections continued to do so while on the pump. And then it dawned on us that the reason they had bad hypos on injections was because they were on too much insulin, and had not been taught how to adjust insulin doses safely. Although everyone who was started on a pump was provided with a few days training, for many this was not just their introduction to the ins and outs of using a pump, but also their first introduction to the concept of carbohydrate counting, ICR, ISF, correction doses and so on. It will come as little surprise then that in many cases, we found that after a year of using the pump, some were still using the same meal time dose for all their meals, and many had never changed their pump settings from when they were first started. Little wonder therefore that many who had hypos on injections also had hypos on a pump, as apart from the means of delivering insulin, nothing else had changed.

This led us to recommend that the teaching on insulin management and carbohydrate counting should be separated out from the training in how to use a pump. Personally, I went one step further, and still do recommend that everyone with type 1 diabetes, who has not already done so, should receive such training, as in many cases this would resolve issues with hypos, etc. After six months they would be reassessed, and only then would a recommendation for insulin pump therapy be made, if despite such education, the person was still experiencing difficulties in establishing good control of their diabetes without hypos. In practice that meant that everyone was asked to attend a BERTIE course, before they would be considered for pump therapy. This also meant that when the time came for them to start a pump, the pump training could focus on ensuring that they understood the principles of using a pump and were properly trained in its use. In 2011, we looked at our data and showed that patients who attended BERTIE prior to commencing pump therapy had less diabetes-related emotional distress and fewer problems with hypoglycaemia. They also had a more sustained improvement in diabetes control once on the pump, and we concluded that attending BERTIE or a similar course helped people be better prepared and better able to benefit from the advantages of using an insulin pump.[44]

In 2008, NICE revised its guidance and provided much wider criteria that qualified individuals for insulin pump therapy. They essentially allowed anyone with type 1 diabetes to start insulin pump therapy if they had difficulty achieving an HbA1c below 8.5 per cent (69mmol/mol). NICE also stated that children under the age of 12 could be started on a pump, although rather bizarrely they said that once they reached 12 they should be switched to injections again if they could manage it. I am not sure this suggestion was ever acted upon; I cannot think of a worse possible time, just as they are entering the uncertainties of puberty, to take a pump away from a young person who may have been on it ever since they were diagnosed with diabetes. Despite these much more generous criteria, many places imposed artificial limits on the number of pumps that could be dispensed in any year, and in some cases the number was laughingly small. In Bournemouth we negotiated with the payer (then called the Primary Care Trust) an annual sum of money to be allocated to insulin pumps, and then negotiated hard with the companies to drive the costs down so that we could squeeze as many new pumps out of the same pot. Although the number of diabetes centres offering pump therapy was increasing, the new guidelines meant that more and more people were eligible for a pump, and an ever-increasing number of patients were being referred to us for a pump. With no extra staff available, this put a heavy strain on our service, such that we just couldn't fit everyone in. The pressure to do so meant that sometimes people were not always provided with the same high standard of training when they started the pump and the time between review appointments began to get longer and longer –

sometimes more than a year. Not surprisingly, we began to see that some people were not achieving the benefit we would expect from using a pump. We therefore took a leaf out of our approach to education and designed a year-long programme of group training for people new to insulin pumps.

Prior to starting a pump, we ascertained that each person was competent in carbohydrate counting and insulin dose adjustment, for example by having attended a self-management programme such as BERTIE. That meant that they had already established the correct basal insulin dose, ICR and ISF and so the initial training over a few days focused solely on teaching the detail of using the pump, and adjusting these parameters when required. This training was programmed to start in groups of four people, at set dates throughout the year.

At the initial training, each person's HbA1c was checked and each was asked to complete the PAID (Problem Areas in Diabetes) score. They were also asked to identify the goals they wished to achieve by starting on a pump. Following the initial training, the groups met again every three months, until nine months after the start. The reviews were used to help individuals solve any problems they were having with managing their pump and to adjust the pump settings as required. We also used the opportunity to recheck HbA1c and PAID scores. At one year after the pump start, individuals were reviewed by one of the consultants to assess progress against their goals and to see if any further changes to treatment were required. By careful coordination and a nifty bit of scheduling (that I took great pride in designing), we were able to provide a vastly superior service to support over 48 people in starting an insulin pump each year. As always, we collected the data on their outcomes and found, not surprisingly, that seeing everyone this regularly was associated with significantly better improvement in HbA1c after starting a pump, with also much less diabetes-related distress.[45]

In the nearly twenty years that I have been involved in insulin pump therapy, we found that many derived benefit from the greater flexibility in daily routines and in social situations that the pump gave them, in addition to stabilisation of blood glucose levels and better sleep with a sense of more energy in the morning.

DECIDING WHETHER TO GO ON A PUMP?

The experience in adapting the Bournemouth pump service to the demands placed upon it has convinced me that no one should be started on a pump in a hurry, or without adequate training before, during and after the pump start. Therefore, if you are having trouble with your diabetes management, I would suggest following the same pathway as outlined below, rather than heading straight for a pump.

1. Ensure you are competent in carbohydrate counting and review your current treatment (basal dose, ISF and ICR) and diet as detailed in chapters 10 to 12.
2. Consider using an automated bolus advisor, as described in chapter 11. The Expert meter is a good half-way house as it is identical to the control set for the Accu Chek Combo insulin pump, and its bolus advisor is the same as that is found in the Accu Chek Insight pump.
3. If you are still struggling to achieve stable glucose control, discuss insulin pump therapy with your diabetes team and the pump options available.
4. Ensure you are provided with extensive training on how to use the pump. This cannot easily be done in a quick visit and will likely take a total of several hours, spread over a few visits. It is important that at the end of it you have a full understanding about how to use the pump.

5. Seek a review and advice on optimising your pump therapy every three months for at least the first year.

Now there may be some people where it is obvious that a pump is the best option, and in such cases the journey from steps 1 to 3 can be speeded up. The most striking case I have come across was of a lady whose child would wake up at random times through the night and run around the house, and the poor mother would have to sit up with, and often run around after the child. When she was on insulin injections, this often led to her developing hypos, which was potentially particularly hazardous to her and her child. With the pump, however, she was able to reduce or shut off her basal insulin completely until the child was safely asleep again, and remain free from the risk of hypos. Pregnancy is another situation, where a fast-track approach to steps 1 to 3 is necessary, for obvious reasons. Steps 4 and 5 are essential however, as I still see people who do not know how to adjust their basal rates, even after using a pump for several years.

So, what are the typical scenarios in which you might benefit from an insulin pump? These can be summarised as follows:

1. Very low insulin requirements: There are some people who are very sensitive to insulin and require very low doses. So much so that even using a pen that can dispense in half-unit increments, does not provide the fine-tuning required. In theory this can be overcome by the use of lower strength insulin such as U40 (40 units per ml, compared to the standard 100 units per ml), although this is not available in many countries. An insulin pump can deliver insulin at doses as small as 0.025 units per hour and therefore provides real benefits to those with high insulin sensitivity (for example, those who require less than 15–20 units a day in total).

2. Dawn phenomenon: This is where glucose values rise during the latter part of the night, usually thought to be as a result of the action of growth hormone. This is more likely to occur in teenagers or young adults, but can occur at any age. Using a split basal dose (see chapter 10) can help, but if this does not solve the problem, then a pump can address this very well because of the ability to increase the basal rate as the night progresses.

3. Differing activity levels: As with the example of the lady who was sometimes up half the night chasing after her child, anyone whose activity levels vary unpredictably will find it very difficult to achieve stable glucose control with insulin injections. Examples include people who work in an office, but occasionally may need to help out with physical work, such as unloading supplies or working in the factory. This group also includes people who participate in sport or intensive physical activity on a regular basis. The sudden increase in physical activity puts them at risk of a hypo. This can be offset by having some extra carbohydrate, but by definition, if it is unpredictable, this may not be readily available; and if it happens suddenly, you might just not remember or have time to eat anything. The dose of an injection of basal insulin will be determined by the usual work pattern, and once injected, you cannot take it away. With a pump, you can reduce the insulin infusion rate or even just stop it for a time.

4. People with needle phobia: For anyone with type 1 diabetes, having a dislike of injections, quite apart from a true needle phobia, can have profound consequences. They will quite understandably try and minimise the number of times they have to perform an injection, sometimes with quite disastrous results for their health as a result of chronically high glucose levels. An insulin pump

means you need to insert a cannula once every two or three days, and for some people this makes good management of their diabetes feasible in a way that giving four or more injections a day would never allow.

5. Before and during pregnancy: As we will discuss in chapter 17, very good and stable control of blood glucose is essential in maximising the chances of a successful pregnancy in a woman with type 1 diabetes. Many centres now offer insulin pump therapy to such women.

6. Injection site problems: People who have had diabetes for many years, and especially those who have injected into the same place for a long time, can develop increased thickness of the fat layer below this skin (injection site hypertrophy – see chapter 5). This can lead to large amounts of insulin getting stuck in this excess fat and not properly absorbed. An insulin pump can help in this situation as it releases very small amounts of insulin very slowly. It is also possible to find new areas of skin that are suitable for a pump cannula to be inserted, but less suitable for regular injections.

7. Hypoglycaemia: This is probably the main reason people start an insulin pump. Some experience frequent hypoglycaemia, perhaps as a result of the problems listed above, or because of erratic absorption of big doses of insulin. In many cases this can be resolved by going through the steps of getting the basal and bolus injection doses right, but some people find they are still prone to bad hypos. Others have experienced hypos in the past and as a result want to run their glucose levels higher than ideal. This fear of hypoglycaemia can lead to devastating consequences as a result of long-term high glucose levels. If this applies to you, the fine-tuning of an insulin pump can help gradually increase your confidence that you can achieve stable glucose control without a hypo.

Undoubtedly, an insulin pump offers many benefits, and you may feel that it would be of benefit for you too. There are, however, drawbacks to using an insulin pump, and while in my experience the vast majority of people started on a pump then stay on it, a small minority do stop it for a variety of reasons. It is important to understand that:

1. An insulin pump is just another way of delivering insulin, and you still need to calculate and give your bolus doses, and adjust your basal rates when appropriate. A pump does not do all this for you, nor does it measure your blood glucose levels.

2. An insulin pump in itself will not stop you having hypos; however, if you can identify why you are having hypos and you know how to make the most of an insulin pump, it can greatly help reduce the risk.

3. An insulin pump must be connected to you continuously, all day and night. You can remove it for up to an hour at a time (for example, to go swimming, play sport or have sex), but then it is essential it is reconnected and a blood glucose check performed in case the level has risen too high.

4. Most pumps are connected to the giving set by means of a fine tube or cannula. If this gets kinked, the flow of insulin can be blocked off, or if the cannula gets pulled, insulin might leak out, causing high glucose levels and possibly ketoacidosis.

5. The cannula and giving set need to be changed every two to three days, otherwise there is risk of infection or of the insulin not being delivered and absorbed properly. If you observe standard precautions then the risk of infection is otherwise very low.

6. Some people worry about the pump becoming disconnected, others just do not like the idea of being attached to it all the time. While most people soon come to realise the benefits outweigh

these concerns, in some they do not, and they cannot get used to wearing the pump.

7. If the pump fails, you need to inject insulin as soon as possible to avoid the risk of ketoacidosis. As the amount of insulin in the body at any one time is very small, if the pump disconnects, or the tubing becomes blocked, the interruption of the insulin infusion will very rapidly lead to high glucose levels and the risk of ketoacidosis.

8. It is essential that you are prepared to carry out regular blood tests, at least 4–5 per day to keep an eye on your control and be assured that the pump is working safely.

9. It is also important to have a supply of 'back-up' insulin which can be injected in case of pump failure.

As stated, in my experience, the majority of people find the benefits of an insulin pump outweigh the negatives, however it is important to be aware of the possible downsides, and to discuss the pros and cons with your diabetes team to help you make your decision as to whether to proceed.

CHOOSING AN INSULIN AND A PUMP

Insulin pumps are usually used with one of the modern rapid-acting insulin analogues. As stated in chapter 3, there is little to choose between these, but as it has been around the longest, there is more evidence on using lispro (Humalog) than aspart or glulisine. One study even showed that using regular insulin such as Humulin S (Humulin R in the US) or Actrapid was no worse than using modern analogues, which is good news for those who are unable to access or afford more modern insulins.[46] My general recommendation when starting insulin pump therapy is to continue with the same insulin that you used for your mealtime injections. If you start using a pump at the same time as you start new insulin, it will be difficult to know which benefits are as a result of the pump, and which are a result of the new insulin, for example.

There are a number of different makes of pump, each with their own features. As these change quite frequently, I will not go into a lot of detail about each one, but rather use some examples to highlight the different types available. The diabetes.co.uk website has a useful up-to-date list of pumps available in the UK at http://www.diabetes.co.uk/insulin/Insulin-pumps.html

Standard insulin pump

The standard pump is a small device that contains an insulin reservoir, the mechanism to pump in the insulin and the controls. It is connected to a cannula via a giving set (plastic tubing). The cannula is a small plastic tube or fine needle that sits beneath the skin, through which the insulin is delivered into the fat below the skin. The pump can be programmed to deliver the continuous basal insulin at different rates through the 24-hour period. Bolus doses are given by 'dialling' in the required dose and pressing the control to deliver it. Most pumps allow for different types of bolus, and some include an automated bolus advisor to calculate the bolus dose required. Some link directly to blood glucose meters. For example, the Medtronic pumps link to an Ascensia Contour meter, and Roche Accu-Chek pumps have their own dedicated meter.

Pumps with separate handset

The Roche Accu-Chek Combo comes with a blood glucose meter that also acts as a remote handset that you can use to control the pump. This has almost the identical appearance and functionality of the Accu-Chek Expert meter, and so if you have been using the Expert meter, you may find moving to the Accu-Chek pump a logical next step. The newer Accu-Chek Insight pump has a handset with a similar bolus calculator but different functionality, looking a bit like a mobile phone. The pump's settings, basal rates and bolus doses can all be controlled via the handset. And as it doubles up as a blood glucose meter, the glucose values are automatically used to help calculate bolus doses. The Dana, Cellnovo and Omnipod pumps also have a separate handset that doubles up as a blood glucose meter.

Patch pump

A patch pump is a miniaturised pump that is worn as a 'patch' adhering directly to the skin. The pump has no controls on it and there is no tubing. The pump is controlled by a remote handset that also acts as a blood glucose meter. The Cellnovo and Omnipod pumps are examples of patch pumps.

Pump with continuous glucose monitor (CGM)

Medtronic is the only company that manufactures both insulin pumps and CGM systems. These are now available in one device. The most advanced models include a suspend function, that automatically shuts off the insulin delivery if the sensor measures or predicts imminent hypoglycaemia. The Animas pumps can link to the Dexcom G4 CGM system, although in 2017 Animas announced that it was withdrawing from the insulin pump market.

Closed-loop system

The holy grail for those in the field of diabetes pump technology is the so-called artificial pancreas or closed-loop system, where the pump automatically adjusts the insulin infusion rate according to the blood glucose level as measured by the sensor. Medtronic now has a pump that includes this functionality as discussed in more detail in chapter 21.

As you might expect, the cost of pumps and their consumables (tubing etc) can vary quite considerably and not all pumps will be available in every diabetes clinic. CGM is not generally covered by the NHS in the UK or by many insurance systems in other countries, however some people opt to have a pump that has CGM functionality and choose to pay for their own CGM equipment.

SETTING THE BASAL RATE

Once you have your pump, you will need to be trained in its use. The first thing to do is to learn how the various buttons and controls work (these are of course different for each model, and are not within the scope of this book). Then the basal rate needs to be set. This is generally done by taking your usual total daily dose of insulin and reducing by around 30 per cent. This is then halved to provide the total basal insulin to be delivered over 24 hours. So, if you were on 40 units in total on injections, this would be reduced by about 13 units to 27, and divided by two to give 14 units as the basal insulin. The 14 units can either be given at a constant rate (in this case, 0.6 unit per hour) or as a variable rate. Some pumps have a system that will automatically convert the dose into a rate that varies according to average requirements during the 24-hour period. Otherwise, your diabetes team can help you vary the basal rate depending on your past experience. For example, if you have experienced the dawn phenomenon, then the rate can be increased during the early hours of the morning; conversely if you have had hypos during the night, the rate can be decreased. To a certain extent, the initial basal rate will have a degree of trial and error and will need to be checked by performing basal profiles to determine that you have the correct basal rates. Thus, do not expect perfect glucose control straight away – the important thing is that when you start the pump you are not getting too much insulin that could cause a hypo, and if your glucose levels rise too high for a while, this is not of too much concern, and is certainly better than having a bad hypo.

Assessing your basal rates is done in a similar way as someone on injections assesses their basal dose. The difference is that as the basal rate can be adjusted hour by hour (or even more frequently), it is preferable if you can obtain more glucose measurements, for example every two hours during the day, and at least one measurement during the night, as indicated on the schedules below and reproduced in appendix 2 on page 335 (you can photocopy this page for later use):

To check overnight basal rate

Eat a normal meal (ideally with less than 80g carbohydrate and without alcohol) by 8pm in the evening and then check your glucose levels at the following times. Have a normal breakfast at 8am:

Time	8pm	10	11	12	1am	2	3	4	5	6	7	8	9	10
Current basal rate														
Glucose level														
Grams carbohydrate														
Bolus dose														

To check morning basal rate

Skip or have a carbohydrate-free breakfast at 8am and a normal lunch at 1pm. Check at the following times:

Time	8am	9	10	11	12	1pm	2	3
Current basal rate								
Glucose level								
Grams carbohydrate								
Bolus dose								

To check afternoon basal rate

Have a normal lunch at 1pm with no carbohydrate until 7pm. Then have a normal evening meal. Check at the following times:

Time	1pm	2	3	4	5	6	7	8	9
Current basal rate									
Glucose level									
Grams carbohydrate									
Bolus dose									

To check evening basal rate

Have a normal evening meal at 6pm with no carbohydrate afterwards and check at the following times:

Time	6pm	7	8	9	10	11	12
Current basal rate							
Glucose level							
Grams Carbohydrate							
Bolus dose							

Note that completing these charts will also enable you to check the bolus doses taken for breakfast, lunch and evening meals according to the time of day being assessed.

Do not try and perform these checks on consecutive days, rather try and complete them over a period of two weeks or so, on days that reflect your normal daily routine. Avoid strenuous exercise on test days and do not perform the basal tests if you have had a hypo in the previous 12 hours.

If you are surprised about the result of a profile, or do not feel it is representative of what normally happens, it would be best to repeat the profile before adjusting your basal rate. If you experience a hypo during a basal profile check then obviously you need to stop the test and treat the hypo as described in chapter 7. Unless there was a clear reason why you went hypo (intense exercise for example), I would advise you immediately reduce the basal rate at the appropriate time to reduce the risk of another hypo, rather than repeating the exercise.

When you are new to pump therapy, I would recommend that you discuss the results of your basal profiles with your diabetes nurse or educator, who can advise on when and by how much to adjust your basal rate. Remember that just as with a basal insulin injection, with these profiles you are looking for glucose levels to be stable (apart from within 2 hours or so after a meal). Over time, you will become more confident in making changes yourself. It is always recommended that you repeat the basal profiles about a week after you have made any changes, to check that they have had the desired effect.

The following examples show some of the patterns you might see:

Time	10pm	11	12	1am	2	3	4	5	6	7	8	9	10
Current basal rate	0.8	0.8	0.8	0.6	0.5	0.5	0.5	0.6	0.7	0.8	0.8	0.8	0.8
Glucose level (mmol/l) (mg/dl)	6.7 121		6.4 115			7.2 130			7.5 135		7.7 139		7.9 142
Grams carbohydrate											25		
Bolus dose											3		

The glucose level rises gradually from 12 midnight until 8am. This suggests that more insulin is needed during this time. Increasing to 0.6 units per hour from 2am to 5am would be a reasonable initial adjustment.

Time	8	9	10	11	12	1pm	2	3
Current basal rate	0.8	0.8	0.8	0.6	0.6	0.6	0.6	0.6
Glucose level (mmol/l) (mg/dl)	6.9 124		6.0 108		5.1 92	4.2 76		
Grams carbohydrate						40		
Bolus dose						4		

Here the glucose level falls gradually between 10am and 1pm and so the basal rate could be reduced to 0.5 from 11am to 1pm.

Time	1pm	2	3	4	5	6	7	8	9
Current basal rate	0.6	0.5	0.5	0.5	0.5	0.6	0.6	0.8	0.8
Glucose level (mmol/l) (mg/dl)	5.1 92		7.3 131		6.8 122		6.7 121		7.5 135
Grams carbohydrate	40								
Bolus dose	4								

The afternoon profile is reasonably stable and the basal rate can be left unchanged at least until 7pm. The evening profile will determine if the rate needs to be changed after that.

Time	6pm	7	8	9	10	11	12
Current basal rate	0.8	0.8	0.8	0.8	0.8	0.8	0.8
Glucose level (mmol/l) (mg/dl)	6.8 122		7.8 140		8.3 149		6.7 121
Grams Carbohydrate	50						
Bolus dose	5						

Although the glucose level rises after the evening meal, this could be a delayed effect of the meal rather than insufficient basal insulin. By midnight the level has returned to a similar level to that at 6pm and so it should be fine to leave the basal rate unchanged during this period.

Most pumps offer the option to have at least 2 different profiles. I generally suggest you start with one basal rate profile at first. You can then add in alternative basal profiles to cater for different situations, depending on your experience. For example, some people find that their activity level is so different at weekends than during the week, that they find it easier to have separate weekday and weekend rates. Others, who participate in long distance running, may choose to have a rate for run days. These can be built up over time, as you gain experience in how your basal insulin needs vary in these different situations.

TEMPORARY BASAL RATES

Your requirement for basal insulin reduces during periods of increased physical activity, and it is therefore important that you reduce your basal rate at such times. This can be done either by removing the pump completely or by applying a temporary reduction in the basal rate. Removing the pump is an option for up to an hour, and is the preferred option for most people while swimming or for contact sports like rugby or American football. Some who partake in sports such as football also choose to remove the pump, although the intermittent high intensity activity of such sports can increase insulin requirements and so there is a risk of an excessive rise in glucose levels. Some choose to remove the pump for sexual activity (see chapter 17). In each case it is important to check the glucose level once you reconnect the pump and give a correction dose if required.

Applying a temporary basal rate reduction is the preferred option wherever possible. With most pumps, this is expressed as a percentage basal rate reduction, so that if you choose a 40 per cent reduction, the rate will be 40 per cent less than the programmed rate, regardless of whether it changes during the period of rate reduction. Thus, if during a two-hour period of a 40 per cent reduction, the rate is 1 unit per hour for the first hour and 1.2 units per hour for the second hour, the reduced rate will be 0.6 units then 0.72 units per hour respectively. A 50 per cent reduction would provide 0.5 and 0.6 units per hour. For anything other than very mild intensity exercise, I would suggest starting with a reduction of between 40 and 60 per cent. Ideally the temporary rate should be applied at least 1–2 hours before you start the exercise, although in practice this may not be feasible, for example when the increased activity is spontaneous or unexpected. I also suggest checking your glucose at the end of the period of activity, before reverting to the normal basal rate, as if it is low you may wish to leave the reduced rate for an hour or more longer.

The basal rate can also be increased for periods when you need more basal insulin. As with injections, these are generally for periods of stress or illness. If you become unwell, and notice your glucose levels are unusually high, then you can increase the basal rate by 30 per cent or more. In some situations, you may need to double the basal rate, however I would not suggest increasing beyond 30 per cent in the first instance, to avoid the risk of hypoglycaemia. You can always add in correction doses if this isn't sufficient. These increased basal rates can be set for up to 24 hours at a time which is helpful if you are unwell for a few days.

In the time before and during menstrual periods, basal insulin requirements can increase and then decrease. Using a pump can greatly help manage this situation, as will be discussed in more detail in chapter 15.

TYPES OF BOLUS DOSE

The flexibility in being able to vary the basal rate is one of the main advantages of an insulin pump. The other is the ability to use different types of bolus dose, to cater for different types of meal. There is the standard bolus dose, delivered over a short period of time, which is essentially the same as giving an injection. The other types of bolus are an extended or square wave bolus, and a dual or multi wave bolus. Different pump companies give these features different names, which can be confusing, but their features are very similar, as described below.

The extended or square wave bolus describes the situation where a bolus is delivered over a prolonged period. So, if you inject 10 units as an extended bolus, rather than it being infused immediately, it can be delivered as a continuous infusion over two hours (i.e. at a rate of 5 units per hour). This is particularly valuable if you are at a party and grazing over a couple of hours, for example. It can also be used when at a restaurant, eating a meal that might take two to three hours, rather than giving separate boluses. The third scenario is when eating a meal with a high total carbohydrate (e.g. more than 80g) and/or high in fat content (such as a pizza) as a lot of carbohydrate will take time to be digested and the fat significantly delays the speed at which the carbohydrate is absorbed. Sometimes it may be necessary to extend the bolus for up to 4–5 hours. The final situation in which this type of bolus is extremely useful is for people who have gastroparesis. This is a condition where the nerves that control the muscle contractions that empty the stomach have been affected by diabetes, and so the stomach empties very slowly. As a result, the absorption of a meal will be prolonged, and so a standard bolus risks causing a hypo as the insulin will start acting long before the food has been absorbed into the blood stream.

The dual or multi-wave bolus is essentially a combination of a standard bolus together with an extended bolus. It actually mimics the body's own pattern of insulin secretion more closely than a standard bolus. It is particularly useful for meals that contain a mixture of fast and slow acting carbohydrate.

Unless you have gastroparesis, in which case it will be helpful to use extended boluses as soon as you start using the pump, I would generally suggest using standard boluses initially. By checking your blood glucose two hours after meals, you will begin to learn which sort of foods might require an extended or dual-wave bolus.

In my experience, an insulin pump provides the best likelihood of achieving near-normal blood glucose levels without hypoglycaemia, particularly in individuals who have varying activity levels. However, I have also seen people who have continued to have very high glucose levels despite having a pump. This emphasises that, as with so much else, the pump will only be effective in stabilising your diabetes control if it is used properly and with the correct settings and in conjunction with frequent blood glucose monitoring.

14

CONTINUOUS BLOOD GLUCOSE MONITORS AND DATA DOWNLOADS

CONTINUOUS GLUCOSE MONITORING (CGM)

Having an accurate idea of your blood glucose is essential if you are to achieve good control of diabetes. The ability to do that has improved beyond all recognition compared to the 'technology' that was available when I first started working in diabetes.

Blood glucose meters first came into widespread use in the late 1980s, and although their performance has improved since then, their basic functionality remains very similar. The next advance was the advent of continuous glucose monitoring (CGM) in 2000. The first CGM devices were produced by MiniMed (now part of Medtronic). They used a sensor that was inserted below the skin, and that recorded the glucose concentration in the interstitial fluid (the fluid between cells), rather than the blood. This was then converted into an estimate of the level in the blood. The first systems were 'blind' to the user. That is, there was no immediate reading of the glucose level; rather, the sensor was worn for three to five days, and then the data downloaded to provide the blood glucose readings over that period. The information was used to identify trends in glucose levels, and was interpreted by a health professional to provide advice on changing insulin doses.

However, the new glucose sensors were not without problems. For a start they were very expensive, and generally only available as part of clinical trials or for specific situations. There were also problems with them not always working very reliably, and finally, logistical issues meant that the patient often didn't get the information from the sensor until well after the sensor had been fitted, by when it was often out of date.

The next advance was the advent of 'real time' glucose monitoring. This for the first time provided the user with a display that showed the glucose level in real time, so the user could react to the level to prevent or treat a hypo or hyper event. This was particularly useful for people who use an insulin pump, as it provided the opportunity to suspend the insulin delivery if the sensor showed the glucose level falling too low. However, the systems were still expensive and generally not available on the NHS or reimbursed by health systems in other countries. Unless people chose to fund the equipment themselves, such systems were (and in many cases still are) only available for those who have a history of disabling hypoglycaemia that persists even with the use of an insulin pump. I have known some people who have had continuous monitoring for this reason, yet found it not particularly helpful. This has been a problem where the sensor appears not to provide an accurate reading, especially if it senses a low blood glucose and triggers an alarm, when in fact the glucose level was within the normal range. However, as sensors become more reliable, so does the prospect of linking a glucose sensor to an insulin pump becomes a step closer to producing what has become known as the artificial pancreas, that we discuss in more detail in chapter 21.

More recent MiniMed pumps have a built-in capacity to double up as glucose sensors (known as sensor-augmented pumps (SAP), and the pumps can suspend the insulin infusion (rather than just give an alarm signal) if the sensor detects a hypo. The latest models respond to the trend in glucose and suspend when a hypo is predicted, with the aim of avoiding the hypo happening in the first place. Although other pumps can link with Dexcom sensors, they do not provide the option of automatically suspending the insulin in response to a hypo. However, this is a fast-changing world and if you are interested in these aspects, I recommend you consult the websites of the companies that produce pumps and CGM systems for the latest available functionality of their products.

In view of the rapid advances being made, whenever anyone has asked me what I foresee to be the next big advance in management of type 1 diabetes, I always say that it will be the routine availability of continuous monitoring, as the technology improves and prices come down. Until then, for anyone who does not suffer from severe hypos, they will have to buy the equipment themselves. I know of many people who have done so and derived benefit, even if they only use a sensor for maybe one week each month, in order to curtail the cost.

In the past few years there has been a further exciting development that is, I think, the start of that becoming a reality. That is the advent of what is known as 'flash' glucose monitoring, in the form of the Freestyle Libre system produced by Abbott. Whereas most continuous monitoring systems require the user to perform blood tests at least once a day to calibrate the sensor, the Freestyle Libre comes ready-calibrated and has been marketed as an alternative to regular blood testing. It is worn as a patch, usually on the upper arm, that holds a glucose sensor inserted below the skin. The sensor records glucose levels every five minutes, and rather than providing a continuous reading of them, the user can read their glucose by placing the reading device over the sensor whenever they want to know their glucose.

This system enables the measurements since the previous reading to be downloaded, allowing the user to see a display of their glucose levels throughout the 24-hour period. It is important to note that, as with CGM systems, the Freestyle Libre measures glucose in the interstitial fluid, which lags somewhat behind the glucose level in the blood. Therefore, the UK DVLA (the body that set rules for driving) requires a standard blood test to be performed before driving. A standard blood test should also be performed at times of suspected hypoglycaemia. Apart from these situations, users do not need to do regular blood tests; each sensor lasts two weeks and costs around £57 (€64, $74), which brings it into reach of being affordable for many people. The reader costs about the same as a one-off cost and contains a bolus advisor that can be used to calculate insulin boluses, according to the measured glucose level and the carbohydrate to be eaten, (in the same way as the Insulinx described in chapter 7). The system is licenced for use in children from the age of four, for whom the availability of such a system is a huge step forward, as it allows parents to check their child's glucose level at any time, without the need to draw blood on a regular basis. Since November 2017, the Freestyle Libre system has been available in the UK, reimbursed by the NHS for selected patients, as determined by each local area. Eligible patients could include those with problematic hypoglycaemia, those who might otherwise need an insulin pump, or those who currently need to undertake finger-prick blood tests each day, because of erratic glucose levels.

DOES CONTINUOUS GLUCOSE MONITORING (CGM) MAKE A DIFFERENCE?

If you are considering using one of these systems, it is important to consider the reasons for doing so and how you feel you would benefit, especially as for the foreseeable future, most people will be paying for it out of their own pocket. There has been a lot of research published over the past few years that provides good evidence of the benefits of continuous glucose monitoring.

Perhaps the best evidence of the benefits of CGM comes from research co-ordinated by the Juvenile Diabetes Research Foundation (JDRF) in the US. They studied over 300 adults and children with type 1 diabetes. They were randomised to either use standard home blood glucose testing, or to use a CGM device for six months.[47] The majority of the participants (around 80 per cent) used an insulin pump, and the rest used injections. The study showed that there was a significant improvement in HbA1c in subjects aged 25 and over who used CGM; they also had more stable glucose control with more levels within the target range of 4–10mmol/l (71–180mg/dl) and no increase in hypoglycaemia compared with those who used standard glucose monitoring. Interestingly, this improvement with CGM was not seen in adults younger than 25 or in children; one possible explanation for this is that many in these groups did not use the CGM device continuously. The study showed that there was a significant reduction in both high and low glucose levels in those using CGM, meaning that so-called glucose variability was much reduced, but only if the CGM was worn more than 4 days at a time.

Most of the early studies of CGM were with people who used insulin pumps. There is now evidence that it is also beneficial for those who use injections. Data from a large US register of people with type 1 diabetes (the TID Exchange Registry) showed that overall, people who used a pump had better HbA1c levels than those on injections. However, when looking at those who also used CGM, there was no difference between the control achieved with a pump or with injections.[48] Another study showed that people on injections who used CGM had an HbA1c that was on average 5mmol/mol (0.5 per cent) lower than those using standard blood testing.[49] This showed that using CGM, the average HbA1c achieved was 63mmol/mol (7.9 per cent) compared to 68mmol/mol (8.4 per cent) using standard blood testing. This research does suggest that access to CGM significantly improves glucose control in people who use insulin injections as well as in those on a pump.

Use of the Freestyle Libre, which is a so-called 'flash' rather than continuous glucose monitoring system also has benefits over standard blood glucose testing. A paper in the Lancet in 2016 reported on 120 people who used the Freestyle Libre and another 120 who used standard glucose testing.[50] Those who used the Freestyle Libre accessed their glucose values on average 15 times each day compared to an average of 6 tests done by the group with standard testing. The Freestyle Libre group reduced the average time spent in hypoglycaemia from over 3½ to 2 hours per day, whereas those using standard testing showed no such improvement. This is a significant benefit from a system that does not produce continuous readings. In the past couple of years, a number of people in the UK have funded the Freestyle Libre themselves and in my experience, may have benefited significantly with less hypoglycaemia or lower HbA1c or both. The greatly reduced number of finger-prick tests is also seen as a great benefit.

The benefits of sensor-augmented pumps (SAPs) have also been demonstrated. SAP is the term that describes a pump that doubles up as a glucose sensor and that stops the insulin infusion when the glucose falls below a certain level. Use of the Medtronic Veo SAP was shown to be effective in reducing the time spent with glucose levels too low.[51] The most recent SAP systems are designed to stop the insulin before the hypo has actually happened, as a result of the system recognising that glucose levels are falling and predicting they will fall too low. If these systems prove to be reliable, they will be particularly helpful for people with reduced awareness of hypoglycaemia and who have problems with hypos at night.

As might be expected, the benefits of using sensor-augmented pump therapy are only seen when the sensors are used continuously. Some people find wearing sensors uncomfortable, or find the alarms unreliable, and so wear them only infrequently. Not surprisingly, this will not lead to the benefits available with SAP and the studies showed that the sensors do need to be worn continuously to derive the advantages of reduced hypos and better control.

DATA DOWNLOADS

One of the features of CGM is that they usually provide a visual representation of glucose levels, either on the device itself, or when uploaded to a display on a dedicated app or on the web. Viewing glucose levels in this way can be very helpful, especially in identifying patterns that occur on a regular basis, such as, for example, a tendency to low glucose levels after lunch. You don't have to use CGM to benefit from such systems.

Most glucose meter, sensor and pump manufacturers have their own programme to display data in different formats. These are often available free of charge to people who use their product. Some produce a standard set of reports that cannot be altered much, whereas others allow much greater flexibility in how data are displayed. These include a simple diary that lists all the glucose results according to date and time. I find this of limited use as it is often not easy to identify patterns. Bizarrely, the tables are often also displayed in reverse date order, i.e. the most recent at the top of the page, which I also find difficult to interpret. To me the most useful are graphs that show the blood glucose levels as a continuous line over several days, and as a graph that shows the glucose levels of each day superimposed on the same graph. The Accu Chek 360 system, produced by Roche, is compatible with most Roche glucose meters and pumps and I find it one of the most versatile currently available.

The following example shows how the Accu Chek 360 can display all the glucose values from an individual for a month, in different ways that are so much more useful than just having the results as a series of numbers in a book or on a screen. Looking at the first graph, you can see that there are some very high and also some low values. You can also see, by looking at the summary data at the bottom, that this person did an average of 1.6 tests each day, which should immediately prompt a discussion about why this was, and what could be done to encourage the individual to do more tests each day. When looking at data like this, I first look to see if there are any hypos, and there are three between the 14th and 18th of the month and then again on the 26th. There are also a couple of near misses on the 6th and the 8th of the month. What all these have in common is that the low values almost all came after high glucose levels. This immediately suggests that the lows could be as a result of a too high correction dose given because of the high glucose level that preceded it. And note how sometimes the low is then followed by another high, perhaps as a result of over-treating the hypo by taking in too much sugar.

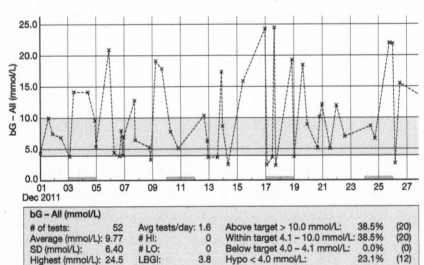

bG – All (mmol/L)					
# of tests:	52	Avg tests/day: 1.6	Above target > 10.0 mmol/L:	38.5%	(20)
Average (mmol/L): 9.77		# HI: 0	Within target 4.1 – 10.0 mmol/L:	38.5%	(20)
SD (mmol/L):	6.40	# LO: 0	Below target 4.0 – 4.1 mmol/L:	0.0%	(0)
Highest (mmol/L): 24.5		LBGI: 3.8	Hypo < 4.0 mmol/L:	23.1%	(12)

If ever you get this pattern of highs and lows, I always suggest you deal with the lows first, which in this case would mean adjusting the ISF (insulin sensitivity factor) to reduce the correction doses. By then avoiding lows, this should help avoid the next high.

The next screen I look at is called the standard day or modal day view. This shows the tests for each day linked together and shown according to the time of day, as in the following example, with the same data as the first graph but in the different format.

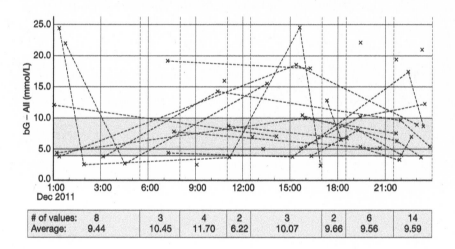

# of values:	8		3	4	2	3	2	6	14
Average:	9.44		10.45	11.70	6.22	10.07	9.66	9.56	9.59

This enables you to see that there is a particular risk of lows during the night. It also shows that the lonely crosses in the top right corner were all high and were on days when no other tests were done (as they are not joined by a line to any other results). This is a very clear demonstration of how missing tests can easily lead to the glucose level becoming quite high by the end of the day.

These systems can also display data on insulin infusion rates and bolus doses from a pump, or on insulin injections given and carbohydrates eaten, if these have been entered into a meter, such as the Accu Chek Expert or Insulinx.

There is also a system called Diasend (www.diasend.com), which is able to display data from most devices. You can create an account free of charge and use it to display the data from your meter, in a similar format to the ones shown here.

Many clinics use these systems to enable you to discuss your glucose data as part of a consultation, and this can be very useful in helping decide if any of your insulin doses (basal dose or rate, ICR or ISF) need to be changed. I know some people also find it very useful to have access to a system at home so that they can view their own data in between clinic visits. These systems can also enable your diabetes team to review your data and perhaps save a clinic visit.

15

DAY TO DAY LIFE AND TYPE 1 DIABETES

We have looked at the complex process required to work out the parameters needed to calculate your bolus insulin doses, and you would be forgiven for thinking things couldn't get any more complicated. But life can be just that – complicated. So here I look at ways to adapt to what daily life throws at you.

Your ICR and ISF should work fine for most situations, when everything is going well. You may even have different values for different times of the day, to account for increased physical activity at certain times of the day, for example. However, when life throws a spanner in the works, your insulin requirements could change quite significantly, and you will need to increase or decrease your insulin doses accordingly. This is much easier to do with an insulin pump, as you can increase or decrease the basal rate with a few clicks on the pump; but if you are on insulin injections you can also make adjustments, although a little more forward planning is an advantage.

ILLNESS

On page 94, we discussed the initial steps to take if you experience high glucose levels while feeling unwell. Please refer to these again, to refresh your memory, as ketone testing is an essential part of managing illness. To recap, if your glucose levels are raised above 14mmol/l (250mg/dl) and you feel unwell, it is important to check for increased levels of ketones in your urine or blood. If ketones are present, then you need even more insulin to correct high glucose levels, and may need to seek medical attention. Even without ketones being present, illness very frequently leads to high glucose levels. In the first instance, you should treat these by adding a correction dose to your bolus doses, as discussed in chapter 11 (see page 133).

Once you get an idea of how much extra insulin you need, you can increase your insulin to carbohydrate ratio (ICR) to prevent the glucose levels rising in the first place. So, for example, instead of taking 1 unit for every 10 grams of carbohydrate, you might need 1.5 units. In some situations, for example if you are unwell for a number of days, it will also be helpful to increase your basal insulin also. If you are on a pump, this can be done by applying a temporary basal rate increase. If you are on injections, you can increase the basal insulin dose. In both cases, the size of the increase will be determined by how high your glucose levels are, and I recommend discussing with your diabetes nurse or educator before making such adjustments. It is not unusual for an increase of between 30 and 50 per cent, or even higher, to be required.

It's helpful to understand why this is. During periods of illness, the body mounts what is called an 'inflammatory response'. That means that the immune system sends out cells and antibodies to attack invading bacteria or viruses. Part of that response also includes the release of hormones such as cortisol (the body's natural steroid) and adrenaline. Part of their actions include increasing the release of glucose into the bloodstream from the liver. In someone without diabetes, the body will also increase insulin secretion to help keep blood glucose levels stable; thus in a person with type 1 diabetes, illness is associated with higher than normal glucose levels, and insulin doses need to be increased to counter that. However, different types of illness can have different and at times unexpected effects on glucose levels. I have often been struck by how relatively minor viral infections, that cause no more than a bit of a headache or runny nose, can be associated with very high glucose levels – and yet other times apparently more serious infections seemed to have little effect on glucose levels. In the former case, it may not be immediately obvious that it is an infection that is causing the high glucose levels. The immune response that causes glucose levels to rise quite rapidly can also shut off equally rapidly, leading glucose levels to fall back down again quickly. And so if you are on injections, and you increase your basal insulin during a period of illness, you need to be aware that your basal requirement might fall quite suddenly, while your last, increased, dose of insulin is still working hard to bring your glucose levels down, increasing the risk of a hypo. Some people just use correction doses of their mealtime insulin to provide the extra insulin required during illness. While not ideal, this is still preferable to just riding out the period of high glucose levels, until the illness subsides. Not only could you feel quite unwell as a result of the high glucose levels themselves, there is a risk that they might actually exacerbate the illness, especially if it is due to an infection. Bugs like sugar, and in addition to antibiotics, fighting them requires that glucose levels are kept under control.

STRESS

Stress is another situation that can cause glucose levels to rise. As during periods of illness, the 'stress hormones', in particular adrenaline and cortisol, are increased during times of stress, and unless additional insulin is given these will have the effect of raising the level of blood glucose. This can last for a few hours, or in the case of prolonged periods of stress, for several days. As with illness, the initial response is to use correction doses and then a higher ICR (insulin to carbohydrate ratio), until things settle down again. For longer periods of stress, the dose of basal insulin can also be increased.

It is also important to be aware that some stressful situations can have the opposite effect, namely of reducing blood glucose levels. I do not think we know precisely why this is the case but my own theory, having spoken to many people with type 1 diabetes who have experienced this effect, is that glucose levels tend to fall during periods of high concentration, in other words, when you are using your brain a lot! Although the brain accounts for only 2 per cent of our body weight, it is jam-packed full of cells whirring away at high speed and accounts for 20 per cent of our energy usage, including up to 50 per cent of the glucose in our system. So if your glucose is in the normal range, say at 5mmol/l (90mg/dl), and you undertake a lengthy piece of work requiring much thought, remember that the brain is going to be using up glucose at a faster rate and that could lead to a hypo. Some people, whose diabetes I have treated, have experienced this occurring during business meetings, and will always take a supply of glucose in with them to avoid a hypo. My own experience of such meetings is that they require you to think fast on your feet and they can be stressful. So, I can well understand people equating the low glucose levels experienced to stress, when in fact the main reason could be just that their brains were using so much glucose.

MENSTRUAL CYCLE

Women of child-bearing age, that is from the time of their first period (called the menarche) until they stop during the menopause, experience rapidly-changing levels of certain hormones, especially oestrogen and progesterone every month. These are necessary to ensure that an egg is available to be fertilised every month, and levels are at their highest towards the end of each cycle, in preparation for pregnancy if the egg released that month is fertilised. If not, levels of oestrogen and progesterone fall sharply at the end of the cycle, associated with the next period.

The high hormone levels towards the end of each cycle have a number of effects that are commonly known as pre-menstrual syndrome. One such effect is insulin resistance, as the high hormone levels work against the effect of insulin. In someone without diabetes, the body will produce more insulin to take account of the insulin resistance; however, in someone with type 1 diabetes, the insulin resistance will lead to higher glucose levels in the blood, unless additional insulin is taken. Once the period starts, the insulin resistance and thus glucose levels return to normal very quickly. Some women do not experience much change in their glucose levels associated with their menstrual cycle, while others see their glucose levels rise quite significantly.

If the changes occur regularly with each cycle and can be predicted, and if your periods themselves are regular, then it is possible, with the help of your diabetes team, to change the ICR and basal dose in the one to two weeks before each period, returning to normal doses as soon as the period starts (or the day before).

However, some people find that the effect of periods on glucose levels is different each time, and others have periods that are not always regular. Some seem to have the opposite effect, where insulin requirements increase during a period. In these situations, it is practically impossible to anticipate when the higher insulin doses will be required, and for people on injections, adding correction doses to mealtime insulin is the best option. However, this is not ideal and women in this situation will often benefit from the flexibility of an insulin pump in providing better glucose control before and during periods. Whatever method is used, it is important to be aware that insulin resistance returns to normal quite rapidly and if insulin doses have not been reduced by then, there is a risk of hypoglycaemia.

THE EFFECT OF ALCOHOL

Alcohol forms an important part of many people's social lives. While excess alcohol is harmful, there is evidence that even small amounts of alcohol are associated with increased risk of some cancers, and in 2016, the UK Department of Health revised their guidelines for safe drinking and now recommend that men and women should have no more than 14 units of alcohol a week, ideally with a number of days without alcohol (one unit is found in a small (125ml/5oz) glass of wine, a single measure of spirit or half a pint of standard strength beer). It is also advised to drink alcohol with meals, rather than on an empty stomach. In the US, women are advised to have no more than 7 drinks a week. Some countries in Europe have higher recommended values, especially for men (35 units in the case of Spain!). This reflects the fact that in truth, no one really knows what is a 'safe' level of alcohol. It is also true that individuals, both men and women, handle alcohol differently, and what may be considered safe for one person could be harmful to another.

It is probably fair to say that if you do keep within the current UK or US guidelines, then your alcohol consumption is unlikely to have a significant effect on your glucose control, especially if the drinks you choose contain little carbohydrate (such as wine or spirits). In the real world, however, we know that many people, including those with type 1 diabetes, choose to drink more than the recommended level, and it is therefore important to know how to avoid alcohol causing problems with blood glucose control.

A number of surveys of young adults with type 1 diabetes in the UK, US and Australia all showed a high prevalence of drinking alcohol. Both overall drinking rates, and the rate of those who drank excessively, were similar to those in the general population.[52] In a sense this is good, in that people with type 1 diabetes are behaving 'normally'. At the same time, it reiterates the importance that people with diabetes understand how alcohol can affect their diabetes control, and how to manage these effects.

The most essential piece of information for everyone with type 1 diabetes is that alcohol has a direct effect of reducing the amount of glucose that is released from the liver into the bloodstream when we are not eating, and especially overnight. This will have the effect of reducing blood glucose levels and increasing the risk of a hypo.

The glucose-lowering effect depends on a number of factors, including:

- How much alcohol has been drunk: the greater the amount, the higher the risk.
- The type of alcohol drunk: drinks that contain carbohydrate (such as beer and cider) will help keep glucose levels up, compared to

drinks with very little or no carbohydrate (such as dry wine or spirits).

- Whether it is drunk with a meal: drinking alcohol with a meal generally slows the rate at which we drink alcohol and the rate at which it is absorbed. The carbohydrates in the meal will also help keep glucose levels from falling too far. However, the glucose-lowering effect of alcohol usually occurs after a delay of many hours, long after the meal will have been absorbed, and if a large number of drinks have been consumed over a long evening meal, then the hypo risk will still be there.

- What else happens that evening: physical activity will also tend to reduce glucose levels. Following several drinks in a pub by a visit to a nightclub for a time of uninhibited display on the dance floor will increase the risk of a hypo, especially if accompanied by some shots of spirits. For some, this might be followed by more physical activity in the bedroom, when you least want to risk having a hypo, (about which more later).

Some years ago, I led a set of experiments to look into some of these factors (not the last one though). We asked six men with type 1 diabetes to stay overnight in a hospital room on two separate occasions. This might seem very sexist, but choosing men only meant that we didn't have to take into account the effects of menstrual cycle in women; unless all women were in the same phase of the cycle, it would have been almost impossible to tease out what was an effect of the alcohol as opposed to changing hormone levels. In the early evening they were given a nice meal (by hospital standards, anyway) and towards the end of the meal they drank the equivalent of about 600ml (20oz) of white wine (depending on their body weight) on one occasion, and water on the other. They then went to bed and had blood taken every hour to measure glucose levels and various other tests through the night. In the morning they had a standard breakfast and further blood tests taken until midday the next day. The aim was to compare what happened after drinking wine compared to water. Interestingly, the effect of wine was to reduce the blood glucose values by about 2mmol/l (36mg/dl) from midnight onwards, increasing to about 3mmol/l (54mg/dl) lower by 7am. What was most interesting, however, is what happened later on. After breakfast, five of the six volunteers had a hypo mid-morning after drinking wine the night before; none had a hypo after drinking water. The blood tests showed that drinking wine reduced the amount of growth hormone that was secreted overnight; this led to both a lower glucose level before breakfast, likely due to the effect of reduced growth hormone in reducing the release of glucose from the liver, and a significant increase in the effect of insulin taken with breakfast.[53]

Now we must remember that this was an experiment in unusual conditions on six men, who drank about three quarters of a bottle of wine and then went to sleep. They may or may not be representative of the general population of people with type 1 diabetes (that also includes women, of course) but it provides some important pieces of information that can be used to provide advice.

This research suggested that drinking anything more than three medium (175ml/6oz) glasses of wine in the late evening will reduce glucose levels after midnight and significantly increase the risk of a hypo in the morning, especially before or after breakfast. Adding physical activity (dancing and/or sex) after midnight would of course further increase the risk of a hypo during the night. How can we turn that into advice?

The first and very clear message is that even this modest amount of alcohol will mean less insulin is needed before breakfast the next day, and I now suggest that people inject at most half of their usual insulin dose for breakfast after an evening of drinking.

The second message is that glucose levels will also be lower during the night and, depending on the level before you go to bed, then you may choose to reduce your evening dose of basal insulin.

For those whose drinking continues into the night, there are some further important messages. Firstly, what to do about the basal insulin injection? It is important that this is not forgotten, as excess alcohol in your system with little or no insulin is the perfect recipe for ending up in hospital with ketoacidosis. Therefore, if you anticipate you will be out until well after the time you would usually take your basal insulin, it might be worth taking it before you go out, even if this is a couple of hours earlier than you would normally inject. Reducing the dose by 10–20 per cent will also help reduce the effect of alcohol in lowering glucose levels during the night.

If your night out will include lots of physical activity, then you will likely need further positive measures to keep glucose levels up. At this time, the worst possible thing would be to have drinks with no carbohydrates, such as shots of spirits. Now is the time to drink beer or cider, or to have sugary mixers with your spirits. If you overdo it and have a high glucose level the next day, this is far preferable to having a profound hypo while under the influence of alcohol, as your recognition of the hypo symptoms will almost certainly be impaired, and others around you may just think you are more drunk than normal which could delay you being given treatment for the hypo.

When you do eventually get home, it is important to check your blood glucose before going to bed. Of course, after a few drinks, memory may be impaired and a degree of disinhibition means some people may take risks they wouldn't otherwise take, and this might include deciding not to check the glucose level. Finally, have something to increase your glucose level before going to bed, unless the glucose level is already quite high (say over 10mmol/l(180mg/dl)). This could be in the form of a sandwich, a portion of fries or a similar readily-available late-night snack.

As with everything else, everyone reacts slightly differently and so it is important that you learn what strategies work best for you when you enjoy a night out. The focus has to be on making sure you can enjoy yourself, while ensuring a few basic checks to keep yourself from having a hypo.

A study from a clinic in London used continuous glucose monitoring to measure blood glucose levels in 17–19 year olds over a weekend, during which they consumed alcohol during one 24-hour period followed by an alcohol-free 24 hours. During the alcohol periods, there was evidence of eating meals before going out and use of sweetened drinks. Although glucose levels were more variable during this period, there was no difference in hypoglycaemia compared to the alcohol-free period, suggesting that these strategies enabled individuals to enjoy themselves while protecting them from the adverse effects of alcohol on their blood glucose levels.[54] Despite this, data from people admitted to hospital reveal that alcohol excess still contributes to a high proportion of admissions with diabetic ketoacidosis or severe hypoglycaemia.

CANNABIS

A study of 158 people with type 1 diabetes in the UK revealed that 28 per cent reported using cannabis.[55] In the UK and in many other countries, possession of cannabis for personal use is a criminal offence. In some countries, the authorities turn a 'blind eye' to its use, recognising that it is used by large numbers of people and that arguably its ill-effects are no worse than those of legal drugs such as tobacco and alcohol. I am neutral on that argument, but given that many of my patients have used cannabis, then I think it is only right to include a section on it here as its use, like that of alcohol, can certainly affect a person's diabetes control.

It does this in two distinct ways. The first is that cannabis, like alcohol, is a depressant, and could make you feel relaxed and less able to concentrate. If you take cannabis, you may forget to take insulin or check your glucose level. The more significant effect of cannabis is to increase appetite, leading to what is described as the 'munchies'. Some cannabis users find they end up eating a lot, and if it includes carbohydrate, that will of course increase blood glucose levels. If you use cannabis and develop a regular pattern of eating, you may be able to safely give yourself a dose of insulin to cover the extra food. If not, it is probably safer to check your glucose afterwards and give a correction dose.

OTHER RECREATIONAL DRUGS

Some people with diabetes may choose to use other recreational drugs, just as in the general population. I am by no means an expert on this topic and as the recreational drugs in use change so frequently, it is not within the remit of this book to provide a comprehensive overview of them and their effects on diabetes. However, if you do take recreational drugs, then there are a few important points to consider.

Most recreational drugs fall into one of three groups – stimulants or 'uppers', depressants or 'downers', or hallucinogens. Stimulants include ecstasy, speed and cocaine and can be very addictive, boosting mood and increasing feelings of well-being. They can cause dangerous rises in heart rate and blood pressure, and when their effect wears off, can lead to depression and mood swings.

Stimulants can lead to loss of appetite and to overactivity, both of which can increase the risk of a hypo. They can also increase risk-taking behaviour, which may mean blood glucose is not checked or insulin is omitted. Thus, the precautions described in the earlier section on drinking alcohol also apply here, especially the need to take regular carbohydrate and to check your glucose levels. In addition, there is a risk of dehydration, and it is important to drink plenty of fluids, approximately a pint an hour.

Alcohol and cannabis are types of depressant. Others include amphetamines and heroin. They cause the brain to function more slowly and can affect concentration, balance and coordination. If you take them you might forget to check your blood glucose or give insulin. Both heroin and amphetamines can reduce appetite – although in some people it is increased, as with cannabis.

Hallucinogens include LSD and magic mushrooms. As the name suggests they can distort perception and cause hallucinations, known as trips. Some can be associated with dangerous side effects including high blood pressure, vomiting, heart attacks and seizures. Their effects can last for several hours during which time a user may omit to take insulin or check glucose levels. It is not surprising that some studies suggest that using recreational drugs is associated with an increased risk of admission to hospital with diabetic ketoacidosis.

This information is adapted from that provided in the Streetwise section of the BERTIEonline resource that provides much more detail on the various drugs and their effects on diabetes.

Dr Adam Pastor from Melbourne, Australia wrote a very good summary of the issues around alcohol and other drugs in type 1 diabetes, and has granted permission for me to reproduce his advice to users in order to minimise the risk of reduce harm:

For all drugs (including alcohol):

Look up the potential effects of the drug on diabetes
Keep account of the amount of drug used
Wear a medical alert ID or bracelet
Always use with companions who are aware of your diabetes

| Increase the frequency of blood glucose measurements |
| Do not omit insulin |
| Snack regularly |
| Carry extra short-acting carbohydrates |
| Discuss alcohol and drug use with your health professional |

Additionally, for alcohol:

| Be aware of the risk of hypoglycaemia during the night |
| Eat carbohydrates before and after drinking |
| Consider reducing long-acting insulin dose. |

TRAVEL

Travelling, particularly on holiday or to visit good friends, can be very exciting. It can also be stressful, especially if one or more of traffic delays, airports or lost baggage feature. As with everything else in life, having type 1 diabetes also adds complexities to travel, and this section is designed to help minimise these for you. Of course, this book can't prevent the hassles associated with travel but hopefully the information that follows will help ensure that your diabetes does not add to the other travel stresses.

The most important aspect of travelling is to ensure that you have enough of all your diabetes supplies with you when you travel. That means, in your hand luggage if travelling by air, and always in a piece of luggage that is easy to reach. Not only is it essential that your insulin, pens or needles and blood glucose testing equipment are available to you at all times, insulin quickly becomes inactive if frozen (which may happen in the aircraft hold) or exposed to very high temperatures. If you are going to stay in a hot climate, will you have access to a refrigerator to store your insulin? If not, you may consider purchasing kits that will keep it cool.

So, at the airport, that means carrying your kit through security. For this, it is advisable to have a letter from your diabetes team that explains you have diabetes and that you need to carry your equipment, including needles, with you at all times.

If you are travelling across time zones, your insulin regimen will have to travel with you. In respect of mealtime insulin, a big change in time zones may simply mean that you have an extra meal (and dose) if travelling westwards, or perhaps one less if travelling east. Basal insulin ideally should be taken at the correct time in your new time zone. Thus, if you usually take your basal insulin at 10pm each night, and are flying from the UK to the US, then you would take it as usual at 10pm the night before you fly, and then at 10pm in your new time zone, after your arrival. That might make for a 30-hour day, with the basal insulin running out during that period, but the additional mealtime dose should make up for that. The exception to this rule is if you are going on a short trip of up to four days, when some people opt to keep their basal insulin injections at 10pm at their home time zone throughout. If the time zone change is very large (e.g. over 8 hours), you may wish to take a small additional dose, perhaps a third of the normal dose, of basal insulin at what would be 10pm in the UK to cover the extra-long day, and then the normal dose at 10pm in your arrival time zone. If you are using a pump, don't forget to change the time within the pump and any linked glucose meter so that they are correct for your new time zone (and back again on your return).

When travelling east, for example from the US to the UK, then you will have a shorter day. I still suggest taking the basal insulin as near to 10pm in your departure time zone as possible, but at a smaller dose (60–80 per cent of normal) to take account of the shorter day. You can then have your normal dose at 10pm UK time on the day that you return. As always it is better to err on the side of caution, and if you are uncertain, given less insulin rather than more.

While travelling you will of course inject for meals as you normally do. Be aware that meals on airlines could be much smaller than you would normally eat, thus requiring a smaller dose. However, you will also need to take into account the likely reduced activity (sitting down for several hours) and any anxiety associated with travel, that might increase your need for insulin, and any alcohol that might decrease it.

While you are away, you will probably need a different amount of insulin than while you are at home. On balance, again I suggest that you reduce your insulin doses by 10–20 per cent as many of the factors that affect your insulin requirements on holiday are likely to mean you need less insulin. These include:

- Hotter weather: a higher temperature means insulin is absorbed more quickly.
- Greater activity: unless you are lazing on a beach all day, you may well be walking around a lot more than at home.
- More alcohol: means less insulin needed
- Different food: if you are used to estimating the carbohydrates in your meals by looking at them, or by being used to standard portions, it may be less easy to know how much carbohydrate you are eating, especially if it is in a form you are not used to. As always, err on the side of caution, and top up with a correction later on if required.

Exceptions to the advice to reduce insulin would include a relaxing beach holiday in an all-inclusive resort, or a cruise where you have ready access to food and choose not to use any of the sporting facilities available.

The website www.diabetestravel.org provides further details on planning travel with diabetes, including a travel calculator. This provides slightly different advice to mine in respect of basal insulin, which just goes to show there are always different ways to do these things.

16

MANAGING PHYSICAL ACTIVITY
WITH TYPE 1 DIABETES

Every time we move, our muscles use up energy that usually comes from glucose. Muscles have their own glucose stores (glycogen) for this purpose and these provide enough energy for 'normal use'. With prolonged physical activity or exercise, the body then makes use of the glycogen stored in the liver and then, after about forty minutes, it starts to break down fat to produce ketones as a source of energy.

The release of glucose from the liver is under the control of insulin. In a person without type 1 diabetes, during exercise, the secretion of insulin from the pancreas is reduced to enable the liver to release glucose into the bloodstream, from where it is taken up by the muscles. With most forms of exercise, there are also other hormone changes, specifically increases in cortisol, glucagon and adrenaline. These all antagonise the effect of insulin, which also helps mobilise the glucose stores into the bloodstream. They also promote the breakdown of fat into fatty acids that are then used to produce ketones. All these changes occur while still ensuring the level of glucose in the blood remains within normal limits.

In someone with type 1 diabetes, however, the pancreas cannot respond to exercise by reducing the amount of insulin. The other hormone changes generally happen quite normally, although glucagon secretion can be reduced in some people with type 1 diabetes. The insulin level will of course be determined by how much has been injected. If too much has been injected, then the liver will not be able to release glucose into the bloodstream, with increased risk of hypoglycaemia. If too little has been injected, then the effect of the other hormones will lead to glucose levels rising too high. That is a delicate balancing act that everyone with type 1 diabetes has to be able to master. It is complicated, as the amount of insulin required depends not just on whether you are exercising, but also the type, intensity and duration of the exercise, as well as the time since the last bolus insulin injection. As everyone varies in their response to exercise, a number of different strategies will be needed for different people. The aim of this chapter is to try and explain the general principles to managing exercise, and to provide you with information that will help you discover what works best for you. (It is such a vast subject that I cannot possibly cover all eventualities for all forms of exercise here, but there are some very useful resources available online that provide much more detail, that I reference later in the chapter.)

We have come a long way from the days of old when people with type 1 diabetes were advised not to participate in sport or other forms of exercise. It is quite understandable how that advice came about: at that time, most people were on one or two injections each day of fixed doses of insulin and blood glucose testing was not available. More recently there have been several examples of world-class sportsmen who have reached the top of their sport while living with type 1 diabetes. These include the Tottenham Hotspur soccer player Gary Mabbutt, the Pakistan cricketer Wasim Akram, the New Zealand cricketer Craig McMillan, the US Olympic swimmer Gary Hall and the Great Britain rower Sir Steven Redgrave.

While you may not aspire to reach the same level of achievement, we are all encouraged to undertake regular exercise, and that includes people with type 1 diabetes. It is usually enjoyable, and that is good for mental health; exercise is also very good for physical health and has distinct benefits for someone with type 1 diabetes. These include reducing the risk of diabetes complications, helping maintain a healthy body weight, improving insulin sensitivity (meaning you need less insulin), lowering blood glucose and also lowering blood pressure and cholesterol levels.

Note that the title of this chapter is 'managing physical activity with type 1 diabetes'. This is very deliberate and is to emphasise that ANY increase in physical activity will likely have a beneficial effect on your blood glucose levels, and so may require you to change your usual diabetes management. From the description above, it will be apparent that if your muscles have to use up more glucose than normal as a result of being a bit more active, then there is a risk that your blood glucose levels will fall too low, especially as the other hormones that will tend to push up glucose levels generally won't kick in at low levels of activity. Of course, all of us use up some energy with moving around every day, and that will help determine how much insulin you need. Thus in chapter 11, when we discussed insulin to carbohydrate ratios, I explained that if you are generally more physically active at work during the day than when at home in the evening, then you will need a lower ICR at breakfast and lunchtime than in the evening. However, if you sit behind a desk all day at work but take the dog for a walk every evening, you will need a higher ICR in the day than in the evening.

INCREASING ACTIVITY IN YOUR DAILY ROUTINE

So, the first thing I would like to cover is thinking about how you can increase your physical activity as part of your daily routine. Our modern-day lifestyles are so different from just a few generations ago, when most people got around by walking or cycling. Our ancestors didn't go to the gym, or go jogging. They kept healthy by using their bodies for the purpose they were designed. Humans are designed to walk, and walking is the most accessible form of exercise for everyone, apart from those with physical disability which makes walking difficult. Hence an obvious target for increased activity is to walk more, and use the car less. The UK Department for Transport estimates that one in five car journeys is less than one mile! Consider setting yourself a target, for example, to use the car only for journeys greater than one mile. That would mean walking to the shop round the corner for that extra carton of milk or the newspaper, rather than driving. If you work within two miles of your home, then consider walking to work. It might be a struggle at first but as your fitness increases, you should find it gets easier, and you will have accomplished significant exercise and saved money.

Cycling enables you to travel faster and further than walking. The UK and the US are both not very cycle-friendly, and although the number and extent of cycle paths is increasing, too often they are an after-thought, sharing a narrow strip of the edge of the road with heavy traffic. This contrasts with countries like Belgium and the Netherlands where cycle paths are the rule rather than the exception. However, cycling is gaining popularity and recent British successes in the Olympics and the Tour de France, as well as cycle-hire schemes in many cities are increasing the trend. Some workplaces are becoming more cycle-friendly too, offering changing and showering facilities as well as secure cycle parking areas. As with walking, cycling to work or to the shops provides excellent exercise.

If your work is further away, consider whether it is possible to use public transport. And if there isn't a bus stop right outside your home or work, so much the better, as the walk at either end will do you good! If there is a bus stop right outside your work, consider getting off at the stop before to increase the walking distance. Do you take children to school by car? Walking with them will not only help your health, it will also benefit them too.

If you must use the car (to do the weekly shop for example), try and increase your walking distance by parking as far away from the shop entrance as you can – and where there are usually lots of free spaces.

Or sell your car. Forty years ago, it was almost unheard-of for families to have more than one car, yet they managed to survive. If a couple shares one car, only one of them can drive it at any one time, which means the other one will have to manage without it. As long as it is shared fairly, they will both necessarily have to engage in more active travel, by walking, cycling or using public transport.

If your job involves long periods of sitting, try and get up for a couple of minutes every hour, in order to break your sedentary time. Are there any tasks you can do standing, rather than sitting? Is there scope to change your job to one which involves more physical activity?

Get a hobby. Learn to play a musical instrument. Even playing the piano consumes calories. Playing the saxophone consumes even more. Both involve movement and the use of various muscles. Both will get you away from the TV or computer, and may even be enjoyable for you and those who listen to you.

Why not join a club? Preferably one which doesn't involve eating or drinking too much. It doesn't have to be a sports club. Anything that will get you involved in an activity is good. Even better if you can walk or cycle there.

In summary, any way in which you are able to increase physical activity and reduce time sitting down within your daily routine will help improve your overall health in many ways. It will also mean you will need lower insulin doses and help maintain a healthy weight.

MANAGING CHANGES TO YOUR USUAL ROUTINE

Now let's look at changes to your physical activity that are not part of your everyday routine. These could include going for a walk, housework such as vacuum-cleaning, shopping, gardening or even having sex. I have met people who have experienced low blood glucose levels as a result of each of these, and other types of increased physical activity. So, the first thing is to be aware that such activities will affect your blood glucose level, usually by reducing it. Once you understand that, you will realise that it is important to know what your glucose level is before you start such an activity. It may be that you have already checked your level, but if not then it would be advisable to do an extra check, just in case it is on the low side putting you at risk of a hypo. Then, it is important to take some action to ensure that the activity will not cause you any problem with a low glucose level. That action will either be to have less insulin, or to eat some extra carbohydrate. There are pros and cons of both as shown in the table below:

	Less insulin	More carbohydrate
Pro	- you do not have to eat extra.	- good for unplanned activity. - can be a nice reward after you have done the task.
Con	- requires planning, so has to be done before the activity.	- risks weight gain if done frequently.

Wherever possible, I advise that you plan such activities in advance, so that you can reduce the dose of insulin you take with the meal beforehand. That requires a degree of forward-planning, for example to decide the night before what activities you will do the following day. Thus, if first thing in the morning you have already decided you will go shopping after breakfast, then you can have less insulin with your breakfast to compensate for the increased activity. I generally recommend a reduction of at least a third. Depending on how much walking you will be doing, you may need to reduce by over a half. So, if your normal insulin at breakfast would be 6 units, you should consider taking between 2 and 4 units.

If, however, you have just had breakfast and your friend calls round on the way to the shops, and you decide to go with him, you will have already had your insulin. Ideally you would wait until after lunch, so that you can reduce your lunchtime insulin, but that probably isn't an option as your friend has already planned to go that morning. So it is important to know that your glucose level is not too low (hopefully you will have checked your glucose before eating but if not it would make sense to check it before you set off), and also to check it after about an hour at the shops. That could coincide with a coffee stop, where you could have a small snack to keep you from going low for the rest of the trip.

Similarly, if you are sitting down after breakfast and seeing it is a nice day, you decide to cut the grass, it would be preferable to do that after lunch, so that you can reduce your lunchtime insulin accordingly. However, if the forecast is for heavy rain at noon, you will want to do it in the morning, which means you will need to take some extra carbohydrate to avoid a hypo.

As a rule I would suggest a snack of between 20 and 30 grams, and ensure that you check your glucose before your next meal so that you can give a correction dose if necessary.

In reality, many of the types of increased activity, while not part of your everyday routine, are routine and will be repeated every so often. This means that you can learn from your own experience to judge how much you should reduce your insulin beforehand, or how much carbohydrate you should take during or after the activity to keep your glucose levels stable.

EXERCISE – MORE STRENUOUS PHYSICAL ACTIVITY

Having ascertained that all physical activity will potentially affect your blood glucose level, we now need to consider when that activity is more intense or sustained than activity that is part of everyday living. And that is how I would define exercise. Although that rather neat definition (though I say so myself) covers just about any type of exercise or sporting activity, that in itself is not enough to tell us how a person with diabetes should manage it. That will depend of the type of exercise (aerobic, anaerobic or a mixture), its intensity and its duration. It will also depend on the time since the last meal or insulin injection, and the blood glucose level at the start of exercise. Let's therefore look at each of these in turn, starting with the last.

1. Blood glucose level

   In view of the risk of hypoglycaemia, it is essential that your glucose level is not too low before starting exercise. It is also important that it is not too high, as this could indicate that you have insufficient insulin in your system. In this situation, hormones such as cortisol and glucagon released during exercise could cause your glucose level to rise very rapidly. A good starting point would be to aim for a blood glucose between 7 and 14mmol/l (125–250mg/dl). As you become more confident in managing your diabetes during exercise, it may be possible to start at a lower level than this. It is also advisable not to undertake strenuous exercise if you have had a hypo within the past 24 hours as you are still in a high-risk period for another hypo, and/or less warning of a hypo. If your glucose level is lower than 7mmol/l (125mg/dl), you will need to take 15 to 20 grams of carbohydrate and then retest after at least twenty minutes to ensure the level has come up. If it is higher than 14mmol/l (250mg/dl) then it is recommended to check for ketones. If these are elevated then you are advised not to exercise and to manage your glucose levels as described in chapter 7. If ketones are not elevated, then a correction dose should be given before you exercise and glucose levels checked regularly during exercise.

2. <u>Type of exercise</u>

Next, it is very important to understand the effect of the type of exercise on your blood glucose level. There are two basic types of exercise, aerobic and anaerobic. Aerobic exercise requires blood to be pumped to the muscles to deliver oxygen to be used during the exercise. This requires the heart rate and breathing rate to increase for the duration of exercise. Aerobic exercise is also known as 'cardio' exercise. The common forms of aerobic exercise include running, cycling, swimming, walking and rowing. Aerobic exercise can generally be sustained for long periods, depending on the fitness of the individual. **Aerobic exercise usually causes the blood glucose level to fall.**

Anaerobic exercise on the other hand is exercise that requires high levels of energy to be available over a short period of time. It utilises systems that use glucose without oxygen, and result in a build-up of lactic acid. The most classical anaerobic exercise is weight lifting, where a high amount of energy is required in the muscles for a short time. Other types of anaerobic exercise include track and field events such as long jump, pole vault and boxing. Aerobic exercise at high intensity, such as sprinting, also become anaerobic. **Anaerobic exercise usually causes the blood glucose to rise**, as it is typically associated with high levels of stress hormones that increase glucose levels.

A number of people with diabetes have told me of their frustration that they have started to exercise to help improve their glucose control, only to see their glucose levels worsen. Often, they have been lifting weights or spinning (cycling at very high intensity) both of which are anaerobic exercise. I advise them to undertake more gentle aerobic exercise, and usually they are very pleased with the effect on their glucose control.

In reality, a number of sports include a mixture of both aerobic and anaerobic activity. These include most team sports such as soccer, American football, rugby, cricket, baseball and basketball. In each of these, there are periods of relatively low intensity exercise (or sometimes none at all in cricket) interspersed with very high intensity exercise. The overall effect on blood glucose will then depend on the relative proportion of time spent in each type of exercise.

3. Intensity and duration of exercise

We have already seen how very intense exercise can become anaerobic and cause glucose levels to rise. Apart from this, as the intensity of aerobic exercise increases, so also does the risk of hypoglycaemia. Long-duration aerobic exercise is also associated with higher risk of a hypo than short duration exercise.

4. Time of last injection

The best time to exercise is when you have relatively low levels of insulin in your system, but not too low. Therefore, early morning (before breakfast) is a good option, so also is the evening, before the evening meal. If you are exercising within three hours of a mealtime insulin injection, or bolus, then it is recommended to reduce that dose according to the intensity and duration of exercise. It is also important to be aware that exercise using muscles in the arms or legs will increase blood flow to those areas, and thus increase the rate that insulin is absorbed. It is generally advisable to inject rapid-acting insulin into your abdomen to avoid this possibility.

Putting this all together, how can you then keep your blood glucose levels stable while exercising? As already mentioned, the first task is to make sure your glucose level is neither too low, nor too high. Next is to adapt your routine by either reducing your insulin as just mentioned, or by increasing your carbohydrate intake before, during and after exercise, or a combination of both.As glucose is the main fuel for muscles, then traditionally athletes (with or without diabetes) have been advised to take high amounts of carbohydrate in preparation for exercise. This has led to the development of ExCarbs,[56] which suggests how much extra carbohydrate should be taken by a person with type 1 diabetes, to minimise the risk of hypoglycaemia. This extra carbohydrate is usually taken before, during and after the exercise and can be done in three ways:

1. As extra carbohydrate

   ExCarbs recommends replacing 1 gram of carbohydrate per kilogram (about 0.45 grams per pound) of your body weight for every hour of exercise. So, if you weigh 80kg (176lb), and will be running for 60 minutes, then you will need an additional 80 grams of carbohydrate. This could be taken as 25 grams at the beginning, 25 grams after 30 minutes and 30 grams at the end.

2. <u>As a reduction in insulin dose</u>

Using the example above, you will need 80 grams of carbohydrate to cover your exercise. You can then use your ICR to convert this to an equivalent insulin dose reduction. Thus if your ICR is 10, you will need to reduce your insulin by 80 divided by 10 = 8 units. If your meal is 100g, then instead of taking 10 units, you would reduce by 8 and take just 2 units.

3. <u>Or as a combination of both</u>

Some people use a combination of reduced insulin and taking some carbohydrate. So in the above example, you could take an additional 40 grams of carbohydrate and 6 units of insulin (10 – 4) with your meal to cover your exercise.

Only you can work out which is the best approach for you. I would generally favour reducing insulin rather than additional carbohydrate and would suggest trying option 2 or 3 first.

As well as an increased risk of a hypo during exercise, there is also a risk afterwards, and sometimes several hours afterwards. This is because once you have stopped exercising, your body begins to replenish its glycogen stores in your muscles and your liver. It is therefore important to have a meal that includes carbohydrates, together with an insulin bolus that may need to be at a reduced dose. If you exercise in the evening, you may also need to reduce your bedtime basal insulin dose.

Some people use the glucose-raising effect of anaerobic exercise to protect them from having a hypo as a result of sustained aerobic exercise. The effect of this has been demonstrated in a number of studies. In one, a single ten second sprint added to the end of 20 minutes cycling at moderate intensity prevented blood glucose falling following exercise compared to when the sprint was not added.[57] In another, a similar effect was seen by adding in 15-second sprints every 5 minutes during a 45-minute period of cycling.[58] So, if you do prolonged aerobic or cardio exercise, then including short sprints can help protect against a hypo.

EXERCISE WITH AN INSULIN PUMP

Using an insulin pump makes it much easier to make the changes to insulin doses that are needed to undertake exercise safely. This is because it delivers basal insulin as a very small quantity of insulin as a continuous infusion, rather than a large dose once or twice a day; furthermore, the infusion rate can be changed at any time, using the pump's controls.

Most insulin pumps can set a temporary basal rate increase or decrease, and this is exceptionally useful to help manage exercise. The insulin infusion can also be suspended altogether for a time. Or the pump can simply be disconnected. This is quite safe for up to one hour, and many people who participate in water sports or contact sports choose to remove their pump. While this is probably necessary for swimming, I generally recommend that the pump be worn continuously and set at a reduced basal rate during other sports, especially those that include an anaerobic element.

In preparation for exercise, or any increase in physical activity, it is recommended to reduce the basal rate between 30 and 90 minutes before starting exercise. I would generally suggest a reduction of 50 per cent initially. With experience you will be able to determine if you need to reduce by more or less than this for any given activity. The basal rate should remain reduced for up to 90 minutes and possibly for several hours, after the end of the exercise period. A reduction should also be made in any bolus doses before or after exercise. Some bolus advisors in insulin pumps or blood glucose meters can be set to calculate a reduction in dose for different levels of exercise.

EXERCISE AND A LOW-CARBOHYDRATE DIET

If you have adopted a low-carbohydrate diet, then you may find the recommendations for exercise conflict with your usual way of eating. One of the most prominent advocates of a low-carbohydrate diet is Professor Timothy Noakes, from South Africa, who was instrumental in identifying the benefits of carb-loading prior to exercise in the 1980s. Despite being an avid runner all his life, he gained weight and developed type 2 diabetes in his fifties. This led him to review his own diet and to embrace a low-carbohydrate diet. However, he still advocates that athletes may need a carbohydrate load prior to exercise, although of 125–200 grams compared to the more normal 500 grams.[59]

By contrast, Dr Ian Lake who blogs at type1keto.com describes how he runs half-marathons on a very low-carbohydrate diet. He does this without any carb-loading or change to his usual insulin dose. His meals are mainly based on protein and fat, and as he only injects rapid-acting insulin when a correction dose is needed, he injects basal insulin only. He finds he does not need to reduce the dose of basal insulin, as the effect of any protein meal before exercise, plus the adrenalin and other stress hormones that kick in as he starts exercise, tend to keep his glucose from falling. He is also able to run having fasted for several hours, without a risk of hypo during or after exercise. His experience at least is that exercise can be managed with much more stable glucose levels on a background of a low-carbohydrate diet and low insulin dose. As exercise is so individual, however, it is important to understand that each person may respond differently to exercise and so may have to adopt their own approach.

Whatever diet or insulin regimen you use, each different type of sport can have different effects on glucose levels and the amount of insulin you require, and it is not possible to provide specific detail on each. Thus, whether you use an insulin pump or injections, it will require some experimentation on your part to find the strategy for managing exercise that works best for you. Remember the top priority is to avoid hypoglycaemia, and so erring on the side of caution is recommended, even if it means glucose levels running high a few times. You can always correct a high glucose, and that is far preferable to suffering a bad hypo during a sports match or while swimming. Seek advice from your diabetes team – they will probably know of other people locally with type 1 diabetes who undertake regular exercise, and a number of internet forums host discussions on the topic. I also recommend you look at the runsweet.com website which has a wealth of information from people on how they manage their diabetes while participating in a range of different sports.[60]

If you are a parent of a child with type 1 diabetes then it can be very difficult to take physical activity into account when determining the correct insulin dose, as children's activity levels can vary so much, and sometimes very unpredictably. Many parents will understandably want their child's glucose levels to run a little higher than ideal, especially if they are on insulin injections rather than a pump and anticipate their child may be quite active, in order to minimise the risk of a hypo.

Finally, I would like to share some reflections on type 1 diabetes and exercise from Gavin Griffiths, a young man who was diagnosed with type 1 diabetes at the age of eight. He now travels the world, extoling the virtues of exercise to children and young people with type 1 diabetes. He also participates in several endurance events, including in 2013 running 30 miles a day for 30 days across the UK. He writes a blog on the diathlete website and here shares some of his experiences:[61]

'When I was first diagnosed with type 1 diabetes as a child, my prime concern was evident from the first question to the Doctor: "Can I still play sports?!" The answer lacked encouragement. It included concern about the risks of hypoglycaemia; risks of potential coma and details to my worried parents regarding the use of glucagon to save their child in a bad hypo. A lot of risk talk. While it is important to understand these risks, an 8-year-old diagnosed with such a self-demanding condition requires one aspect above all else: positive reassurance. This seemingly negative change to life all but shattered my childhood confidence. However, my passion for sports and exercise became the key factor of finding myself again – and learning a lot about managing type 1 diabetes in the process!

With type 1 diabetes, it is not so much the type of sport that determines how your blood glucose levels will be affected, it is the occasion and types of movements you will take on within the sport. For example, a goalkeeper on the football field will probably experience a different effect on their blood glucose levels from a midfield player, especially after the game. An early personal experience that showed me how blood glucose levels could rise during exercise came in the form of a childhood street fight. With 'hypo' shakes occurring, my unpleasant opponent kicked my energy drink over whilst mocking me. Now you do not mess with someone when they are hypo! As the fight went on – in a stop-start, almost round-by-round type of street brawl – the energy levels clearly picked up. By the time the fight had finished and I returned home, my blood glucose had risen to quite a high level.

The liver's reaction in releasing stored glucose into the bloodstream, as I experienced during that fight, is influenced by adrenaline. Anaerobic bursts of energy are associated with

*higher adrenaline levels and raised blood glucose levels, whereas
consistent aerobic movements decrease the blood glucose. Recently
I returned from a Global Tour of 5km runs, jogging with young
people with type 1 diabetes around the world. I was not going
full out – and so moved at a more aerobic pace that usually
decreased blood glucose levels. On the other hand, when I have
raced in 5km events and increased the pace to finish sprinting,
my blood glucose levels increase.*

*As a teenager, I played for a semi-professional football
team. After the match, my blood glucose had often spiked quite
high. Lowering the amount of carbohydrates at breakfast and
taking a shot of bolus insulin at half-time became my routine
to prevent high glucose levels during the game. However, after
the match, in which I had endured 90 minutes of exercise, there
was often a delayed crash in blood glucose levels and so I would
eat an earlier high-carbohydrate dinner with less bolus insulin
than usually required for the meal. This post-exercise effect will
differ according to the sport. A Usain Bolt with type 1 diabetes
sprinting 100m in under 10 seconds will experience less of a
decrease in blood glucose afterwards than a Mo Farah after a
10km race.*

*I now run ultra-endurance challenges, aerobic to the core!
Basal insulin is the key; too much basal in the system means a
major hypo threat – especially when out running 30 miles a day
for 30 days across the UK. No basal at all means high glucose
levels. My long-distance regime consists of finding the balance
that suits my body from timing the basal injection, reducing the
dosage according to the extent of the challenge and consuming
the appropriate level of carbohydrates each hour (usually via
tablets) to work with my basal dose.*

*Ultimately, living with diabetes does make playing sport even
more interesting!'*

17

SEX, CONTRACEPTION AND PREGNANCY

This chapter aims to cover all aspects of sex and reproduction that are relevant to both men and women with type 1 diabetes, although some aspects affect one sex more than the other.

Before getting into the details, I thought I would start off by reiterating the information in chapter two about the chances that a child of a parent with type 1 diabetes also develops the condition. Different studies provide different figures, but as a guide, any child of a mother with type 1 diabetes has about a 3 per cent chance of developing it. The risk is slightly higher (5 per cent) for a child born to a father with type 1 diabetes, and significantly higher (20 per cent) for children where both parents had type 1 diabetes. There is an 8 per cent risk in a child whose brother or sister has it. This compares to about 0.1 per cent risk in a child with no immediate family members affected.

This shows the influence of genes in increasing the risk of developing type 1 diabetes but also reiterates than even if both parents have type 1 diabetes, there is only a one in 5 chance that a child will develop the condition. In other words, if two parents both have type 1 diabetes and they have five children, on average only one of those children will develop type 1 diabetes. Therefore, while some people with type 1 diabetes may choose not to have children because of their own health or for other reasons, concern about passing diabetes on to the next generation is not a bar to having children for most people.

SEX

Now obviously for a pregnancy to happen, there has to be sex. And as we discussed in previous chapters, sex is a form of physical activity, and therefore might require a greater degree of forward planning than for people without diabetes. This could include reducing your night-time basal insulin in anticipation, for example. Of course, spontaneous sex does happen, works very well and is possible – it does however carry a risk of hypoglycaemia, and so having a supply of carbohydrate at your bedside to take before, during or afterwards is a good idea. One of the best resources I have come across that discusses this aspect is the section 'lets talk about sex' on the website run by beyondtype1, a US-based charity that supports people with type 1 diabetes.[62] As they very nicely put it, type 1 is the third partner in a sexual encounter, and needs to be treated with respect by both the other partners.

As we discuss further in the next chapter, sex is one of the bodily functions that can be affected by diabetic neuropathy or nerve damage. While erectile dysfunction is well known as a complication of diabetes in men, it is less recognised that women can also experience sexual problems as a result of neuropathy. So, a man may need to plan ahead and take Viagra or a similar drug to help him achieve an erection. There have been claims that these medications can also help sexual dysfunction in women, although none has been licensed for that use. Women may also need lubrication and an understanding partner to help her overcome the difficulties of dryness and reduced genital sensitivity that can result from nerve damage.

FERTILITY

For pregnancy to happen, in addition to sex, both partners need to be fertile. That is the man has to release sperm, and the woman an egg, and they have to meet in the right circumstances. While some studies have shown sperm quality is reduced in men with type 1 diabetes, I am not sure that this is a significant issue. Indeed, we are constantly hearing how sperm counts are reducing in the general population. However, even with these reductions, men generally release millions of sperm each time they ejaculate and it only needs one to get to the egg to make a baby. However, a small percentage of men with diabetes have a condition called retrograde ejaculation, where the sperm are fired the wrong way – into the bladder. This makes it very difficult to achieve pregnancy naturally, but there are techniques available to retrieve sperm from the urine (or directly from the testicle) to be implanted by means of a form of artificial insemination.

Type 1 diabetes in itself does not affect fertility in women, although in women who have very high glucose levels, ovulation (that is, the release of an egg every month) can be affected. This is usually associated with lack of periods, and is probably a good thing as it protects both the woman and baby from the risks of a pregnancy with very high glucose levels. For most women, including those who have moderately-raised glucose levels, ovulation works normally and so becoming pregnant is rarely a problem.

Having said that, for a woman with type 1 diabetes, having a baby is much more complex than for someone without diabetes. This is because high glucose levels at any stage during pregnancy can cause potentially serious problems for the baby as well as for the mother. This is particularly true for the first few weeks of a pregnancy, which is when the major organs of the baby are formed. High glucose levels at this stage can increase the risk of abnormalities or congenital malformations. It is therefore recommended that women strive to achieve very tight control of their diabetes before even conceiving. And that, of course, means using an effective means of contraception and carefully planning the pregnancy. It also means discussing your plans for pregnancy with your medical team, which in any other situation would be very strange indeed.

CONTRACEPTION

So, unless a woman with type 1 diabetes has planned pregnancy, to the extent of working with her diabetes team to achieve stable control of her diabetes (generally an HbA1c of 6.5 per cent (48mmol/mol) on two successive tests at least three months apart), then contraception, or abstinence, is necessary.

In the past, women with diabetes were advised not to take the most common form of pill (that contains both oestrogen and progesterone), as it is associated with an increased risk of blood clots. However, the general consensus is that the risk of an unplanned pregnancy with high glucose levels is much greater than the risk of taking the pill. As with anyone else, the risks associated with the pill are higher if you smoke, have raised blood pressure, have a history of a blood clot such as a deep vein thrombosis (DVT), or a disorder that makes your blood more liable to clot. If any of these apply, then alternatives include using the progesterone-only pill (or mini pill), condoms (male or female) or an intrauterine device or coil. Each has their advantages and disadvantages, and the choice should be based on what works best for you and your partner. Contraception should be continued until you and your diabetes team have agreed that it is safe for you to embark on pregnancy.

PRE-PREGNANCY COUNSELLING

Advice on the impact of pregnancy on diabetes and vice versa should be part of the routine management of all women with type 1 diabetes of child-bearing age. In truth it is not always done very well but as a minimum should include:

- asking if you are taking contraception;
- asking if you are planning pregnancy in the near future;
- advising that diabetes control should be optimised to achieve HbA1c of 6.5 per cent (48mmol/mol) or less before pregnancy, in order to minimise the risks of miscarriage or congenital abnormalities;
- advising of the risks of embarking upon pregnancy if your HbA1c is above 10 per cent (86mmol/mol).

Further details can be found in the NICE guideline on management of pregnancy in diabetes.[63]

If you have not received such advice, the following section briefly covers the risks and what can be done to reduce them.

To me as a seasoned and sometimes cynical medical practitioner, the fusion of a sperm and an egg, the combination of their DNA, the development of an embryo and growth of the foetus into a tiny human being are all quite remarkable. I find it quite amazing that this all happens, in the vast majority of cases very successfully, and all in the space of nine months between conception and childbirth. Although science has advanced our understanding of quite how this all happens, there are still many gaps in our knowledge and I suspect there will be for some time to come.

However, a successful pregnancy doesn't just happen by chance. It happens because nature has designed the human body to function in a way that enables a successful pregnancy to happen. That requires just the right balance of nutrients, hormones and other factors to enable all these processes to happen at the right time and at the right pace. One of these factors is the level of glucose in the mother's bloodstream, as this will directly affect the glucose in the developing baby's blood. Other important factors include the mother's blood pressure, and any medications that she may be taking that could affect any of the developmental processes in any way.

From this, it will be apparent that having type 1 diabetes could easily disrupt the correct balance that is required for successful pregnancy. And that is why it is so important that blood glucose control is as normal as possible throughout pregnancy. All the evidence shows that women with type 1 diabetes who have near-normal glucose control throughout pregnancy achieve the same success rate as women without diabetes.

The reason why the glucose level at conception is so important is because the baby's organs are formed very early on. An embryo of just six weeks already has eyes, ears, heart, liver and limbs in the early stages of development. By eight weeks, all the major organs have been formed. Thus, women who have high glucose levels during this period are at greater risk of having a baby with a malformation. Common types of abnormality include those that affect the heart and the spine (known as neural tube defects, such as spina bifida). Other problems include cleft lip and palate. While some of these (such as cleft lip) are relatively easy to correct, others are much more complex and could affect the health or even the survival of the baby.

Of course, these types of problems occur in babies born to mothers without diabetes. In fact, amongst the general population, around 2 per cent of babies have a developmental abnormality of some sort. This is about the same as the rate for women with type 1 diabetes, whose HbA1c is around 5.5 per cent (37mmol/mol) when they become pregnant. However, for women whose glucose levels are higher than this, the risk of such problems increases. One study showed the risk of abnormality is slightly higher at 4 per cent when the HbA1c at conception is 7.6 per cent (60mmol/mol). However, the risk increases significantly to 10 per cent when the HbA1c is 11 per cent (97mmol/mol) and to 20 per cent when the HbA1c at conception is 14 per cent (130mmol/mol).[64] Pregnancies in women with high glucose levels are also associated with a higher risk of miscarriage, pre-eclampsia (a condition that causes high blood pressure and kidney problems), premature delivery and also increased risk of death of the newborn baby. High glucose levels can also cause the baby to grow too large, to the extent that problems can arise during childbirth and a Caesarean section might be necessary.

From this, you can see that if a woman with high glucose levels has an unplanned pregnancy, there is a high rate of an abnormality or other problem. On the other hand, if you work with your diabetes team to achieve good glucose control, these risks will be very similar to someone who does not have diabetes. That is why it is strongly recommended to use effective contraception to prevent an unplanned pregnancy.

For most couples, planning a pregnancy usually involves discussion between the woman and her partner, and rarely anyone else. It is after all one of life's private decisions in which only two people need to be involved. Often, no one else, not even close family members are told about the planned pregnancy, until the pregnancy is well underway. Not so if you have type 1 diabetes. Once you and your partner have decided you want to try for a baby, the first thing you need to do is contact your diabetes team. Their job is to see you quickly and to support you in preparing for pregnancy. According to the 2015 NICE guideline, this should include:

- empowering you to have a positive experience of pregnancy and childbirth by providing information, advice and support that will help to reduce the risks for both you and your baby;
- explaining that good blood glucose control before conception and continuing this throughout pregnancy will reduce the risks we have discussed;
- giving you and your family members information about how diabetes affects pregnancy and how pregnancy affects diabetes.

Practically, the first step is to make an up-to-date assessment of your diabetes and how you are managing it. That will include measurement of HbA1c, review of your home blood glucose readings and a check on your weight and blood pressure. You should also have a check on your kidney function (blood and urine test) and an assessment of your eyes, if this has not been done within the past six months.

If there is evidence of eye or kidney disease, then this will need to be carefully assessed, as pregnancy can potentially affect either. For reasons that are not completely understood, pregnancy can cause advanced retinopathy to progress, and so it is essential that any necessary treatment is provided before pregnancy. Pregnancy also demands more from the kidneys, which have to handle a greater amount of fluid than previously; pregnancy can be associated with higher blood pressure, and this can also adversely affect the kidneys, especially if there is evidence of some diabetic kidney disease. There are a few situations, in which a woman may be advised against pregnancy, and one of them is advanced diabetic kidney disease. However, if your eyes and kidneys are healthy then there is unlikely to be a problem.

You may need support in optimising your blood glucose control. Now is a good time to review your basal insulin dose (or pump infusion rates), and your ISF and ICR. This in turn will require you to be checking your blood glucose on a regular basis. Some diabetes centres offer insulin pump therapy to women during pregnancy, however, there is little evidence that starting with a pump is of benefit, unless there are other reasons why a pump may be helpful (such as hypoglycaemia during the night or associated with physical activity). I am also not sure that the lead up to pregnancy is the time to embark on such a big change in treatment for your diabetes. There is no need to change your insulin, as all apart from the newest insulins have been used safely for many years during pregnancy.

So far, this section has concentrated on all the things that can go wrong during pregnancy so I feel now would be a good time to emphasise that despite the increased risks, I have looked after many women over the years through pregnancy. Yes, some have had problems, but the overwhelming majority have done extremely well. Many women who previously struggled to get their diabetes under control, somehow manage to summon up whatever it takes to really manage their diabetes well when they become pregnant. However, it does require a high level of discipline in respect to blood testing and insulin management to achieve this. It may also require closer attention to diet. Just as women without diabetes may make a conscious effort to improve their diet, stop smoking or stop drinking alcohol during pregnancy, so you too may feel motivated to cut out some of the less healthy foods that we all enjoy eating from time to time. You may also consider reducing your carbohydrate intake as a means of helping improve your glucose control. A study from Denmark published in 2016 found HbA1c in early pregnancy was closely associated to the quantity of carbohydrate eaten; those who ate less carbohydrate had lower HbA1c levels. This study also found that women who ate frequent snacks tended to have a higher carbohydrate intake and more weight gain during pregnancy.[65]

It is also recommended that in this period, blood glucose monitoring is increased to include some measurements of glucose levels after meals. This is the best way of assessing whether your ICR is correct, and will quickly alert you to the need to make a change, either to take more insulin – or less carbohydrate.

There is also a need to review medications. Some medications that are routinely used in diabetes are not recommended in pregnancy and these include ACE inhibitors and angiotensin receptor antagonists (such as ramipril or losartan) that are used as treatments for blood pressure and diabetic kidney disease, and statins for raised cholesterol. Your diabetes team will be able to prescribe alternative blood pressure medications until after the baby has been born. Folic acid at a dose of 5mg daily is recommended to be started before conception and until week 12 of pregnancy, as this has been shown to reduce the risk of neural tube defects (such as spina bifida). Most diabetes centres will make provision to see you at regular intervals during the preconception period to help you make the changes outlined above and to achieve an HbA1c of 48mmol/mol (6.5 per cent). This process can take several months, and so it is good to advise your team of your plan for pregnancy as soon as you have made the decision. Once you have achieved the desired goals, you will be advised to stop using contraception, and try for a baby.

MANAGEMENT DURING PREGNANCY

Inform your diabetes team once you have confirmed that you are pregnant as they will want to see you as soon as possible, ideally in a joint diabetes antenatal clinic, where midwives and obstetricians are also present. You will need to attend this clinic every one to two weeks throughout the pregnancy. This is so that the obstetric staff can monitor the development of the baby with regular ultrasound scans, while the diabetes team monitor your diabetes and advise on any changes to your treatment. There will also need to be reassessments of your eyes and kidney function at the start of pregnancy and again during pregnancy if any abnormalities were found.

Insulin requirements change significantly during pregnancy; it is important to continue frequent blood glucose monitoring throughout the nine months. You may find you need more insulin during the first few weeks, but then often the insulin requirement decreases until about 16 weeks. It is important that you are aware of this, as it can cause unexpected hypoglycaemia. From 16 weeks, insulin requirements increase progressively until week 37, before reducing prior to delivery. During the latter stages, insulin doses may need to be increased almost daily to keep up with the body's increased need for insulin. It is not unusual for insulin doses to double during pregnancy, and usually the mealtime doses need to increase more than the basal dose.

DELIVERY

It has been established that the safest time to deliver the baby of a mum with diabetes is between 37 and 39 weeks. This reduces the risk of the baby growing too big and also reduces even further the small risk of a stillbirth. In many cases this will require labour to be induced by medication, or for a caesarean section to be performed, if indicated. The delivery date will be discussed with you well in advance, as well as any additional treatments that might be necessary, depending on your own situation.

As soon as the baby is delivered, your insulin requirements will fall rapidly, and it is therefore usual that insulin is given via a continuous infusion that can be adjusted as necessary. If you are on an insulin pump, you should continue with this during labour; if you have insulin injections, these will usually be replaced with an intravenous infusion during labour.

After the delivery, your baby will be checked by a paediatrician to ensure he or she is healthy. In some situations, they may need to be looked after in a special care baby unit for a short period of observation. If your glucose levels have been high during the latter stages of pregnancy, there is a risk that the baby may develop hypoglycaemia after birth and so his or her blood glucose will need to be monitored. Breastfeeding soon after delivery and at regular intervals will help prevent hypoglycaemia.

Soon after delivery, you will be established back on your usual insulin treatment. All mums are encouraged to breastfeed, and this may mean you need less insulin than before the pregnancy and so continued regular monitoring of glucose levels is required.

Once you go home, you will gradually adjust to life with a baby. After what will seem such a long time focusing on your diabetes, your new focus of attention will be the new addition to your family. It is only natural, therefore, that less attention is paid to your diabetes. In the early weeks, and especially while breastfeeding, it is important to avoid the risk of hypoglycaemia, and that sometimes means that blood glucose levels rise a little too high. However, it is important to try and stay on top of your diabetes, despite the additional demands on your time and your attention. At the very least, it is essential that you continue to monitor your blood glucose frequently, so that you know that you (and indirectly your baby) are safe.

In due course, you will be seen again in the diabetes clinic, and your medications can then be reviewed, particularly if any had to be changed for the pregnancy.

18

LONG-TERM COMPLICATIONS AND HOW TO AVOID THEM

The term 'complications of diabetes' generally refers to the long-term effects that diabetes has on various parts of the body. At their worst, these can lead to blindness, kidney failure and amputations. Unfortunately, many people have experienced relatives with diabetes who have been affected in this way. Others will have had the experience of well-meaning friends tell of the person they knew who became blind and lost both legs as a result of diabetes. And on hearing such stories, it's tempting to become fatalistic, and not put the effort into controlling diabetes, on the basis that such complications are inevitable.

Nothing could be further from the truth. Yes, type 1 diabetes can be associated with nasty complications. However, we know that the risk of developing complications is closely related to how well diabetes is controlled. Put simply, if your glucose levels are always high, and your HbA1c is above 85mmol/mol (9.9 per cent) then you have a high risk of developing complications. On the other hand, if your HbA1c is around 50mmol/mol (6.7 per cent) then the risk is greatly reduced and that is why I have gone into so much detail in this book to help you achieve as near-normal glucose levels as possible. Having said that, it is important to understand that the complications of diabetes do not arise overnight, or as a result of a few weeks' high glucose levels. It is estimated that it takes at least five years for advanced complications to become established, and so a few weeks or even months of high glucose levels are unlikely to lead to lasting damage. It is in people whose glucose levels have been high for years that the risk of complications is greatest.

In this chapter, I will describe the common complications of diabetes and how they come about. More importantly, I will also describe what you can do to help prevent them occurring in the first place. My aim is to provide reassurance that they are not inevitable and that they can be prevented. And even in cases where they do occur, if they are picked up early, they can be treated so that they do not develop and cause serious problems.

VASCULAR DISEASE

Most of the complications of diabetes are due to vascular disease, that is damage to blood vessels. These are commonly divided into large and small blood vessels. Large blood vessels are the tubes which carry blood from the heart to all parts of the body (the arteries), and back from the parts of the body to the heart (the veins). The heart pumps constantly to maintain blood pressure, to keep it flowing through the system. As the arteries reach out across the body, they divide into smaller and smaller branches, until they form very small blood vessels called capillaries. It is here that the nutrients contained within the blood (such as oxygen and glucose) leave the blood vessels and enter the tissues they supply, to be used as energy by the cells within the tissue (for example a muscle). It is a bit like a domestic central heating system, where the heart is like the boiler – creating the pressure, the blood vessels are like the copper pipes – carrying the hot water around, and the radiators are a bit like the capillaries – where the energy is transferred to heat the air. However, the analogy then begins to fall down, as in the body capillaries also collect waste products such as carbon dioxide from the tissues to be recycled. Household radiators don't yet do that.

Just as the pipes in the central heating system can get furred up, leaky or blocked, so can the blood vessels. Indeed, when we are born, our blood vessels are beautifully smooth and clean inside, and as we grow older the insides begin to fur up with cholesterol and other substances which form atheroma, or narrowing of the arteries. If the narrowing becomes critical, then the part of the body supplied by that blood vessel will be deprived of oxygen and other essential nutrients. If the blood vessel then becomes blocked completely, then the tissue it supplies will be damaged, and part of it may die to be replaced by scar tissue. If this occurs in a coronary artery in the heart, it is referred to as a heart attack; in the brain, it is called a stroke. A blockage of an artery in the leg may lead to tissue damage in the foot. The process is the same, but the effect depends on which artery is affected.

You will be aware that heart attacks and strokes do not only occur in people with diabetes – they are actually quite common in our society. There are a number of factors which increase the risk of these problems occurring. These include having a family history of such diseases, being overweight, cigarette smoking and having high blood pressure or a high cholesterol level.

Now, there is not much you can do about your family history, however everyone can have a go at stopping smoking and losing weight, and if successful this will significantly reduce the risk of vascular disease, even in people with diabetes.

Whereas large blood vessel diseases can occur in people without diabetes, small blood vessel disease is more specific to diabetes. This is because it generally results directly from the excess of glucose in the bloodstream. Over time this causes small blood vessels (capillaries) both to block off or to become leaky. While this process will occur to some extent all over the body, its main effects are seen in two key areas – the eyes and the kidneys.

DIABETIC EYE DISEASE – RETINOPATHY

Diabetic eye disease (known as retinopathy) is probably the most common complication of diabetes, and also the most studied. This is because it is possible directly to see and document the damage to the blood vessels. The image below is a photograph taken of the back of the eye through the pupil. It shows the retina (the lining of cells inside the back of the eye) which is orange in colour. The capillaries fan out from the optic disc to supply blood to all parts of the retina. These are seen as smooth, fine, red lines. After many years of high glucose levels, these capillaries can become irregular (leaving tiny red dots poking through the surface) or begin to leak (leaving

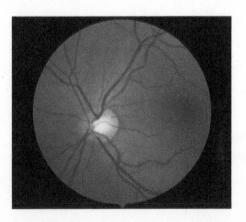

red or white blots). This is known as background retinopathy, or early non-proliferative diabetic retinopathy, which does not affect eyesight. Over time, however, damage to a capillary can cause the area of retina it serves to be starved of oxygen and glucose, and this can change the appearance of the retina. This stage, known as pre-proliferative retinopathy, also does not adversely affect eyesight.

There are two types of retinopathy that do affect vision. The first is a progression of the process described above, where the damaged retina sends out signals to stimulate the formation of new blood vessels to supply the area covered by the defective capillary. This may seem like a good thing, but unfortunately these new capillaries have a tendency to grow forwards into the vitreous (the jelly which fills the eyeball) and they are also are very fragile. This means they have a tendency to bleed into the eyeball, and it is this that can cause blindness.

The other type of sight-threatening retinopathy is maculopathy. This is where retinopathy affects the central part of the retina – the macula. As this area is used for central vision, any damage will affect your ability to focus on what you are looking at. This will make it difficult to read or drive a car, for example, even though the surrounding areas of retina may be relatively unaffected.

As retinopathy can become quite advanced before it affects the eyesight, it is essential that everyone with diabetes has regular screening for retinopathy. This entails having a photograph taken of the back of the eyes, and is described in more detail in the 'Regular Health Checks' section on page 272. The good news is that if retinopathy is picked up early, then treatment is available to stop it progressing to the stage where it can affect vision. Laser therapy is the traditional form of treatment, where a fine laser beam is passed through the pupil to the areas of retina affected. It works by stopping the damaged retina producing the chemical signals which lead to the formation of new blood vessels, and can also help shrink down any which have already formed. It is very effective in preventing blindness.

Recently, newer treatments have become available to treat maculopathy. These are given by injection through the front of the eye into the macula. They are a class of drugs known as anti-VEGF (vascular endothelial growth factor) and can be very effective in protecting vision, particularly when the macula is swollen (macular oedema). They have also been used successfully in cases of proliferative retinopathy, although their effect is often short-lived.[66]

The other piece of good news is that retinopathy can be prevented by maintaining good control of diabetes and blood pressure, and by stopping smoking. While very mild background retinopathy is actually quite common in people with longstanding type 1 diabetes, sight-threatening retinopathy is almost unheard of in those whose diabetes is well-controlled.

DIABETIC KIDNEY DISEASE (NEPHROPATHY)

The other part of the body which is particularly affected by small vessel disease is the kidney. The kidneys are essential organs which help maintain the correct balance of chemicals, salts and water in the bloodstream. As the heart pumps blood around the body, it passes through the kidneys, which sit on either side of the back, just below the ribs. Whereas in most tissues, capillaries transfer nutrients to the surrounding cells, the reverse occurs in the kidneys. Here, specialised capillaries transfer waste products into tiny tubes called collecting ducts. These then lead into the ureter, which takes the waste (urine) into the bladder.

Take glucose for example. When the level of glucose in the bloodstream rises above about 10mmol/l (180mg/dl), the kidneys try and get rid of the excess glucose by removing it into the urine.

This glucose has to be dissolved in water (otherwise you would pee sugar lumps) and so the kidneys release extra water into the urine. This has the result of making the person pass more urine, which in turn makes them dehydrated, which in turns makes them thirsty so that they drink more fluid and keep well-hydrated. So the common symptoms of high glucose levels – excess thirst and urination – are the result of the kidneys doing their job in trying to restore more normal levels of glucose in the blood.

The kidneys act a bit like a filter or a fine sieve, which allows only certain things through into the urine. When the capillaries in the kidney are damaged, the filter becomes leaky (or the holes in the sieve become larger) and this allows substances (such as proteins), which normally should be kept in the bloodstream, to leak out into the urine. Hence finding protein in the urine can be a sign that kidneys have been affected by diabetes.

Just leaking a little extra protein in the urine is itself of little consequence. However, over time, diabetic kidney disease can cause the pressure within the kidneys to rise, which can increase their leakiness. Kidneys are also important in controlling blood pressure, and damage can cause blood pressure to rise, which in turn can increase the pressure in the kidneys so further causing damage. Eventually the kidneys can become further damaged and even scarred, making them less effective in maintaining the correct composition of the blood. This eventually leads to kidney failure and the need for dialysis or a kidney transplant.

Fortunately, just as with diabetic eye disease, this severe form of kidney disease is increasingly rare, and with good care, kidney disease can be prevented. The message is the same: keeping good control of diabetes and blood pressure will avoid these problems. It is important to have a urine test once a year to check if there is the earliest sign of protein leaking into the urine, and if there is, treatments are now available which can help reverse this leak and keep the kidneys healthy. Even people whose kidney function has been badly affected by diabetes can lead long and active lives, thanks to treatments that control blood pressure and prevent any further damage. The commonest such treatment is a class of drugs called ACE inhibitors (such as ramipril or lisinopril for example). They reduce the pressure within the kidneys and as a result can reduce the leak of protein into the urine, helping maintain good kidney function.

And as with eye disease – prevention is better than cure. Keeping good control of blood glucose levels and blood pressure will keep the kidneys working well, even after having diabetes for many years.

DIABETIC NEUROPATHY – NERVE DISEASE

If the blood vessels are a bit like the heating system in your house, the nerves are a bit like the electrical wiring, providing information (sensation) from all parts of the body and power to all the muscles of the body. In fact, nerves are specialised cells whose function is to transmit tiny electrical currents from one end to the other, so they do in fact act a bit like electrical wires.

Sensory nerves have specialised endings in the tissues, which pick up particular sensation. So, for example, if you step on a sharp object such as a pin, nerve endings in the skin will transmit the pain sensation up your leg, up the spinal cord and to the brain. While pain itself is unpleasant, this acts as a protective mechanism for the foot. Within the brain, nerves will connect to the area which controls speech, so that you may exclaim 'ouch' or something less polite. They will also connect to motor nerves, which travel back down the spinal cord, and down to the muscles in your leg, which contract to lift your foot away from the painful object. Sensory and motor nerves control just about every function in the body, from the beating of the heart to the movement of the gut; sweating, sexual function, emptying the bladder and just about everything else are controlled by different types of nerves.

In diabetes, nerve function can be affected by high glucose levels, both in the short term and in the longer term. The short-term effects can be likened to a toxic effect of glucose on the nerves. So it is not unusual, for example, for people to describe tingling in the feet, or of difficulty getting an erection, during periods when their glucose levels are high, and for these symptoms to improve once glucose levels stabilise. In the longer term, more permanent nerve damage can occur as a result of high glucose levels. There are a number of possible mechanisms for this, and it is likely that the accumulation of glucose within the nerves causes direct damage, as well as nerves being affected by damage to the small blood vessels which supply them.

The longest nerves tend to be affected first, and in most people these are the nerves to the feet, followed by those to the hands. As a result, the most well-known type of neuropathy affects the sensory nerves in the feet. This can lead to tingling and gradually to loss of sensation so that the feet become numb. The risk here is that stepping on a pin will not be felt; this in turn may lead to the pin being stuck in the foot, allowing infection to set in, causing ulceration and more extensive damage to the whole foot. If there is also large vessel disease affecting the circulation, then such injuries can be very difficult to heal, and this combination can in some cases lead to the need for amputation.

As every part of the body is supplied by nerves, then many different body functions can be affected by diabetic nerve damage. One of the most common is difficulty getting erections in men, for which treatments such as Viagra can be very helpful. A less common problem is retrograde ejaculation, where damage to the nerves that control ejaculation can lead to semen flowing backwards into the bladder rather than out through the penis. Sufferers experience little or no ejaculation and a tell-tale sign is that the next time urine is passed, it is cloudy because of the semen it contains. This is not harmful in itself, although some people experience pain during ejaculation. What is most significant is that as sperm also pass into the bladder, fertility is greatly reduced. I have known a few people in this situation, where sperm were able to be retrieved and used for artificial insemination, with good results.

There is also extensive evidence that sexual function in women can be affected by nerve damage, commonly resulting in vaginal dryness, reduced sensation and difficulty in achieving orgasm. While men nowadays are much more open is discussing sexual problems, probably because of the availability of treatments such as Viagra, in my experience, women are less likely to mention such problems during a consultation (possibly also because I am a man). Nevertheless, if you are affected in this way and require help or advice, please do speak to someone in your diabetes team about it.

Diabetic nerve damage can also affect the sweat glands, causing excessive sweating, sometimes while eating (this is called gustatory sweating, and thought to be due to the nerves that control salivation getting mixed up with those that control sweating). Effects on the bladder can cause frequent urination or difficulty in passing water; there are medications available although sometimes this may require the insertion of a permanent catheter. The gut can also be affected to cause problems such as heartburn and constipation. More extensive damage can lead to a condition called gastroparesis, where essentially the stomach muscles are paralysed. This means that food is not pushed though the stomach into the gut. As a result food can remain in the stomach for a very long time, causing feelings of fullness and sometimes frequent vomiting after meals. It also causes the delayed absorption of food that requires mealtime insulin to be injected later than normal, and often well after the meal, in order to avoid a hypo. In some cases, a pacemaker can be fitted to the stomach to stimulate the muscles to contract and push the food down.

There are no treatments which can delay or reverse nerve damage and so, as with other types of complication, the key is to prevent it in the first place, by maintaining good control of blood glucose levels. It is important to have feet examined at least once a year, and more frequently if there is any sign of nerve damage. Hopefully there will never be any problems, but at the first sign of any sensory problems, it is important to take very great care of the feet in order to minimise any more extensive damage. Details of the specific treatments available for other nerve problems are shown in the table.

Drugs used to treat symptoms of neuropathy

Symptom	Cause	Treatments available
Erectile dysfunction	Damage to nerves to penis	Sildenafil (Viagra), tadalafil (cialis), vardenafil (levitra) Caverject injections
Excessive sweating	Damage to nerves to sweat glands	oxybutynin
Heartburn	Reflux of acid into oesophagus	Antacids Omeprazole, lanzoprazole
Regurgitation of food	Stomach not emptying properly	Domperidone, metoclopramide
Diarrhoea	Disordered gut motility, overgrowth of bacteria in gut	Codeine phosphate. Short course of antibiotic (e.g. tetracycline)
Constipation	Loss of sensation in lower bowel	Standard laxatives e.g. lactulose, senna

Symptom	Cause	Treatments available
Painful symptoms e.g. shooting pains, pins and needles	Hypersensitivity of nerves carrying pain sensation	Duloxetine, amitriptyline, pregabalin, gabapentin
Frequent urination	Bladder irritability	A number of preparations including oxybutynin, solifenacin, tolterodine
Difficulty passing urine	Loss of bladder sensation	Bethanecol chloride; catheterisation
Fainting, light-headedness	Low blood pressure	fludrocortisone

INFECTIONS, SLOW HEALING AND ORAL HEALTH

Just having diabetes, however well controlled, is associated with an increased risk of infections and increased inflammation. This is because bugs like glucose and thrive in a more sugary environment. This is particularly the case if your glucose levels are high as you will excrete glucose into your urine, which becomes a perfect breeding ground for bacteria. Thus women in particular are prone to urine infections. For the same reason, both men and women with diabetes have an increased risk of developing recurrent thrush if their glucose levels are high. In men this can cause inflammation of the head or glans of the penis, known as balanitis. It usually responds in the short term to standard treatments with antifungal cream or tablets, but will likely return as long as glucose levels are high. Sometimes thrush becomes so entrenched that a long course of antifungal tablets (up to six months) might be needed.

Having diabetes is also associated with changes to the immune system, which can mean the body doesn't always react as well as it should do to infections or to injury. Thus you may have noticed that if you cut yourself, the wound can take longer to heal and be more likely to get infected than before you had diabetes, even if your blood glucose levels are quite reasonable. This is normal. Healing will take place, you just need to be extra vigilant to keep the affected area clean and look out for any sign of infection.

Many people, with or without diabetes have poor gum health. This generally results from the build-up of dental plaque that contains bacteria, causing inflammation of the gums (gingivitis). Left untreated this can affect the bone beneath the gums and lead to the loosening and loss of teeth. For the reasons above, the bacterial infections and gum inflammation can be more pronounced in people with type 1 diabetes, increasing the risk of more advanced gum disease, especially in those with long term high glucose levels. Regular brushing of the teeth and flossing can help reduce the risk. Use of an electric toothbrush with fluoride toothpaste is recommended. Like many of the other complications of diabetes we have discussed, gum disease can occur without you even knowing about it. One sign of gum disease is bleeding from the gums after flossing or brushing the teeth. I have been told that even some dentists can miss it, if they just focus on the teeth. It is tempting to put off going to a dentist, if your teeth seem fine and you do not have any toothache. However, just as with an annual eye examination, please make sure you see a dentist at least once a year, and ask them specifically to look for any signs of gum disease.

SOFT TISSUE PROBLEMS

Finally, there is a group of problems caused by the thickening or stiffening of soft tissues, such as tendons and ligaments, as a result of the effect of high glucose levels. They can affect any part of the body but commonly occur in the shoulder to cause 'frozen shoulder'. This is where the range of movement at the shoulder is limited and painful. It can be treated by steroid injections and sometimes requires to be manipulated or 'loosened up' under anaesthetic.

Another common problem is carpal tunnel syndrome. The carpal tunnel is at the front of the wrist and is where a number of nerves and tendons pass through a narrow 'tunnel' formed by the bones of the wrist at the back and fibrous tissue at the front. As these tissues thicken, they can squeeze the nerves to cause tingling, pain and sometimes weakness in the fingers. Thickening of tendon sheaths in the palm of the hand can lead to Dupuytens contracture, which causes some of the fingers to become flexed so that you cannot straighten them. Both these problems can be helped by surgery to remove the excess tissue.

Discussion of the long-term complications of diabetes is not easy, as to be frank they are not very pleasant. However, I do believe it is essential that everyone with diabetes knows about them, and understands the importance of achieving good control of glucose levels in preventing them occurring. It is also important to set these complications into context and to be aware that great advances have been made in our ability to prevent them and to treat them, and that with appropriate support it is perfectly possible to live a long and happy life with type 1 diabetes with no significant complications.

REGULAR HEALTH CHECKS

In addition to working to achieve good glucose control, avoiding complications also requires each person with type 1 diabetes to have the regular check-ups which are designed to detect the earliest signs of any problems so that these can be treated and in some cases even reversed.

It is suggested that these checks are performed regularly, usually once a year, to assess whether you have any sign of complications which might need treatment. The aim of this section is to explain each of those checks, and how you go about getting them done.

Eye checks are important to detect the earliest signs of diabetic eye disease. To recap, this is usually in the form of abnormalities to small blood vessels. Diabetic eye disease can be controlled, and even reversed, by good control of blood glucose and blood pressure. However, in its early stages, diabetic eye disease does not affect eyesight and the only way of knowing whether you have it is by having a photograph taken of your retina. In the UK, there is a comprehensive eye screening service which is free of charge for people with diabetes. Unfortunately, this is not the case in many other countries, where it can be quite expensive to have the test done, or it might not be readily available. A diabetic eye check is separate from the usual eye test that you might have to determine if you need glasses, for example. The test firstly involves drops being put into your eyes in order to dilate the pupil (to make it bigger so that there is a good view of the retina behind it). You are then asked to sit still in front of a specialised camera, which takes a picture of your retina through the pupil. The image is generally ready very quickly and in many cases, the person taking it will be able to show it to you. In any case, I would encourage you to ask to see it, as it is your retina! Although the operator may be able to give an informal opinion of the image, it will then be transmitted to a grading centre, where it will be assessed by an expert for evidence of any diabetic eye disease. Once that has been done, you will receive a letter confirming the findings. If all is well, there will be no problem, and you will be invited back for another test after one or sometimes two years. If there is evidence of mild, or background, retinopathy, then you will be advised of this and a further test may be recommended in six or twelve months. In the meantime, it would be good to consider what you can do to ensure your glucose levels and blood pressure are as well controlled as possible. If, on the other hand, the image shows evidence of more severe retinopathy, then an appointment will be made for you to see an eye specialist (ophthalmologist) who can perform a more detailed examination and discuss possible treatments with you. Meanwhile, the most important thing is to turn up for the eye test. Some people have told me how they are fearful of having the test done, in case it shows some evidence of diabetic eye disease. While I can understand that fear, I would urge you not to let it stop you having the test done as, in the early stages, good control of blood glucose levels can stop retinopathy progressing and even help reverse it. For more advanced disease, treatment is available which can keep it under control and to protect eyesight.

Just as a regular eye examination is important, so is an examination of your feet. Feet can be affected both by diabetic nerve disease – causing numbness, so that you lose sensation in your feet – and also by blood vessel disease, which reduces blood flow. Both these problems can lead to breakdown of the skin, causing an ulcer. This in turn can lead to infection in the tissues under the skin or in the bone. Poor blood supply can make it difficult to eradicate infection, and cause the need for amputation.

Throughout this book, I have tried to emphasise that developing type 1 diabetes no longer means that that you will inevitably get more and more health problems. However, it is important to be aware of how diabetes can affect health, in order to know how to stay healthy. And in respect of feet, it is important to know how severe and how quickly these problems can occur. I have, for example, experienced how a person with neuropathy can quickly develop an ulcer as a result of wearing shoes that are too tight. In some cases this can lead to deep-seated infection requiring long periods in hospital, and even requiring amputation.

Unfortunately, once blood vessel disease has set in, it is largely irreversible, especially when it affects the small blood vessels. Although there is some evidence that specific forms of diabetic nerve disease can improve with good control of diabetes, this may not be enough to avoid future problems. So, the important thing to emphasise with respect to feet, is that it is essential to prevent problems occurring in the first place.

We have already discussed how good control of blood glucose can reduce the risk of complications. This is especially important in anyone who already has evidence of blood vessel or nerve disease, in order to minimise any damage resulting from these problems. This is why it is so important that your feet are examined on a regular basis, and at least once a year. The examinations are relatively simple, and include a check on the pulses in the feet, preferably using a Doppler machine which assesses the flow through the arteries. The other check is a simple test of sensation, using a nylon fibre called a monofilament, which is used to touch the sole of the feet in specific areas, to see if you can feel it. These tests may pick up problems before you are aware of any change, and if they do, should prompt a review of your diabetes management to ensure that everything is being done to minimise any further damage. These tests will generally be performed by the team at your doctor's practice, or at your diabetes clinic. It does not really matter where the test is done – the important thing is that it is done.

Kidney function is assessed by means of a blood test and a urine test, which should be done once a year. The blood test is to measure the estimated glomerular filtration rate (or eGFR), which measures kidney function. The eGFR is calculated using a formula which depends on the amount of creatinine in the blood. Creatinine, in turn, is a by-product of the breakdown of protein, which is excreted by the kidneys. If the kidneys do not work properly, then creatinine is not excreted into the urine and the amount of creatinine in the blood accumulates. An eGFR above 60 is considered normal. A level below 60 is definitely indicative of some impairment of kidney function. The blood test should be performed at least once a year.

The other test of kidney function is a urine test to assess the amount of a protein called albumin in the urine. Just as the kidney should normally excrete creatinine into the urine, it should not excrete albumin as this is required in the blood. Hence there is normally only a very small amount of albumin in the urine. However, in diabetic kidney disease, the capillaries become leaky, which means that substances such as albumin leak through into the urine. While this is not a good thing, it does provide a simple means of checking whether the kidneys are working properly. All this test requires is that you collect a sample of urine which is then sent to a laboratory to have the levels of albumin and of creatinine measured. The result is expressed as the albumin to creatinine ratio (or ACR for short). A level of up to 3.5mg/mmol or 30mcg/mg (as it is expressed in the US) is generally considered normal. If your result is higher than this, it does not necessarily mean that you have diabetic kidney disease, as there are a number of other factors which may cause a higher level, for example a urine infection or physical activity. My general recommendation is that if the result is raised, then two further urine samples should be taken first thing in the morning. Very often these will be normal, however if the levels are consistently raised, then this suggests that the kidneys have been affected by diabetes.

A slightly raised level – such as up to 30mg/mmol or 300mcg/mg – is termed microalbuminuria (literally, 'small amount of albumin in the urine'). If you are diagnosed with microalbuminuria, you will usually be prescribed medication to reduce the pressure within the kidneys. The usual treatment is an ACE inhibitor, such as ramipril, which is also used to treat high blood pressure (as discussed in chapter 19). This, together with better control of glucose and blood pressure, can help reduce the albumin leak, sometimes to normal levels.

Higher levels of ACR are termed macroalbuminuria. This will also require treatment with an ACE inhibitor. This may not improve the albumin leak, but will usually prevent further damage. Without treatment however, diabetic kidney disease can progress to cause scarring of the kidneys, high blood pressure and eventually kidney failure. Fortunately, this is now rare in people with type 1 diabetes. However, as there are no symptoms associated with albumin in the urine, as with the other checks mentioned in this chapter it is so important to get the urine test done so that if there is evidence of diabetes affecting your kidneys, appropriate treatment can be started in order to prevent more serious damage.

OTHER HEALTH CHECKS

The other checks required are of blood pressure and a blood test to check cholesterol levels (as discussed in chapter 19), which can be done at the same time as the eGFR blood test. Sometimes other tests will be added, such as a check on thyroid hormone levels (an underactive thyroid is a very common problem which can make it difficult to lose weight) or a test for coeliac disease. Like type 1 diabetes, this is an autoimmune condition that affects the lining of the gut, and means you cannot absorb food properly. It is more common in people with type 1 diabetes and can cause problems with hypoglycaemia or weight loss. Blood tests can determine if an individual is at increased risk of coeliac disease, but it can only be diagnosed by having a biopsy of the duodenum (the first part of the small bowel, at the end of the stomach). This is usually done by a procedure known as a gastroscopy, where an endoscope (a long tube through which the operator can see the inside of the stomach and bowel) is passed through the mouth, down into the stomach and into the duodenum.

It is quite common for these annual checks to be done together, as a form of annual review. Ideally you should have all the results available so that you can discuss them with your diabetes team to ensure that you understand their significance, and can then participate in decisions about the need for any treatment or lifestyle change. This is a process that is called care planning. National guidance suggests this should be a collaborative process, in which the person with diabetes plays a full role. My hope is that the knowledge you have gained by reading this book will enable you to do just that.

19

KEEPING BLOOD PRESSURE AND CHOLESTEROL UNDER CONTROL

In chapter 18 we discussed the possible complications of diabetes and how high blood glucose can contribute to these. High blood pressure and high cholesterol levels are also associated with increased risk of complications, and high blood pressure in particular can make some complications, such as eye and kidney disease, worse. This means it is essential to keep blood pressure and cholesterol levels as normal as possible.

While high blood pressure or high cholesterol may be partly due to genes you have inherited from your parents, there is evidence that high insulin levels directly lead to high blood pressure and cholesterol levels. In type 2 diabetes, the body produces high levels of insulin to try and keep blood glucose levels under control, and the high insulin levels probably explain why so many people with type 2 diabetes also have high blood pressure and cholesterol levels.

It is also important to understand that many people with type 1 diabetes also have high insulin levels, especially in what is called the peripheral circulation, that is the blood vessels that go around the body to supply muscles and skin for example. This is because of the need to inject insulin below the skin so that it can enter the bloodstream. This is in contrast to people whose pancreas produces insulin, most of which is in the portal circulation – the blood vessels around the gut and the liver – with relatively little insulin in the peripheral circulation. This is one reason why blood pressure and cholesterol levels tend to be higher in people with type 1 diabetes, and that in turn helps explain why problems such as heart attacks, foot disease and strokes can be more common in people with diabetes.

Now if you choose to adopt a low-carbohydrate diet, this will mean that you need lower insulin doses and that will mean the insulin levels in your blood will be lower than if you eat a lot of carbohydrate. In theory, this should also mean that there will be less of a tendency to high blood pressure, high cholesterol level or weight gain, all of which I see quite commonly in people who have had type 1 diabetes for some time. And with weight gain also comes insulin resistance, which means their blood glucose levels go up, and they need even more insulin.

This is very similar to the situation that occurs in people with type 2 diabetes, and in some cases has been described as double diabetes; that is features of weight gain, insulin resistance, high blood pressure and high cholesterol in people with type 1 diabetes. There has not been much research done on this topic, but I would estimate that this is far more common than many of us realise. As people with type 1 diabetes have the ability to control their insulin levels (by controlling their carbohydrate intake) it is possible that maintaining a low-carbohydrate diet will help prevent some of the problems related to high blood pressure and high cholesterol in type 1 diabetes. Nevertheless, regardless of the diet you choose to follow, it is essential that your blood pressure and cholesterol level are checked on a regular basis.

So, what is blood pressure? It is exactly what it says – the level of pressure that the blood is under in the blood vessels. The cells which make up the various parts of the body need glucose, oxygen and many other substances in order to work effectively. The job of the blood is to carry these substances to all parts of the body. Blood is also the means by which hormones such as insulin, produced in the pancreas, are transported to different parts of the body where they are needed to perform their action (in the case of insulin, to enable glucose to enter muscle cells, for example).

For blood to function effectively, it needs nice clean blood vessels to flow through and it needs to be under pressure, in order to flow. Obviously if there were no pressure, the blood would just sit where it is, like a stagnant pool. The blood pressure comes mainly from the heart, a specialised muscle which contracts to act like a pump, squeezing the blood through the arteries. The kidneys also have an important role in controlling blood pressure, both by regulating the amount of water in the blood vessels, and by producing hormones which help control how tight the blood vessels contract (to increase pressure), or how they relax (to reduce blood pressure). It is evident, therefore, that diseases of either the heart or the kidney may cause problems with blood pressure regulation – and may make a blood pressure problem even worse.

So, you can see that a vicious circle can develop whereby having type 1 diabetes increases the risk of high blood pressure; this combination in itself can then lead to heart and kidney problems; these (especially the kidney problems) can then make the blood pressure problem worse, thus making further complications such as a stroke or heart attack more likely, and so on.

Blood pressure is usually measured using an automated machine connected to a cuff, which is placed tightly around the upper arm. The cuff is then inflated until the pressure around the arm is high enough to stop the blood flowing through the main artery, called the brachial artery. The pressure is then gradually decreased until the flow is returned to normal. As it does, a sensor detects when the cuff reaches the level of the pressure in the arteries while the heart is contracting (called systolic blood pressure), and then the level of the pressure when the heart is relaxing (called diastolic blood pressure). These are then displayed on a digital display as two numbers, for example 120/80, with the systolic pressure first.

So, what should your blood pressure be? There are many guidelines which specify ideal levels of blood pressure in different circumstances, but as a general rule, it should be below 135/85. If you are young, or have evidence of kidney disease or eye disease, then a lower level may be recommended. Now, it is important to mention that, just like blood glucose, blood pressure levels vary quite considerably during the day according to what you are doing and experiencing. In fact, blood pressure can rise very quickly, for example, if you get a sudden shock, or undertake sudden, intense exercise. Just as a single blood glucose measurement cannot give an accurate overview of your diabetes control, neither can a single blood pressure measurement be used to determine your blood pressure control. Ideally, blood pressure should be measured in a relaxed environment after at least five minutes' rest. Yet very often it is measured in a busy clinic setting, perhaps after you have been waiting – and getting more tense – for some time. Some years ago, when home blood pressure monitors began to become more widely available, we checked the blood pressure readings of a number of people with diabetes taken in our clinic, at their family doctor's practice and at home. It came as no surprise to us to find out that the highest readings were those taken in our clinic, and the lowest readings were taken at home, with those taken by the family doctor somewhere in between. So, if your blood pressure is found to be high at a clinic visit, it is probably worth having it re-checked at your doctor's practice, or better still, to purchase a monitor so that you can check your blood pressure yourself. (Again, some years ago we evaluated the accuracy of inexpensive home blood pressure monitors and found them to give similar readings to the much more expensive device used in our clinics.)

I therefore recommend that anyone with diabetes, whose blood pressure has been found to be higher than ideal, buys a machine for home use. These can be purchased from as little as £20 ($26, €22). I would suggest checking your blood pressure no more than once every two weeks, just to reassure yourself, and your doctor, that all is well. Obviously if your blood pressure is high, or you are on medication for blood pressure, then more frequent monitoring may be required.

If your blood pressure has been found to be high consistently, then you are at increased risk of further health problems. It is therefore important to try and reduce your blood pressure. It may well be that you need tablets to achieve this, and we will discuss those later. First, however, there may be some lifestyle changes that will help.

Being overweight and inactive is associated with raised blood pressure. So, losing weight by modifying your diet and increasing your physical activity as described in this book, will also have an effect in reducing your blood pressure. However, there are other specific factors which can affect blood pressure, and these are stress, alcohol and salt.

Stress is part of life – it cannot be avoided. When we are under stress, the body produces a number of 'stress hormones' which gear us up for 'fight or flight', that is to engage in a fight or to run away. Part of the actions of these hormones is to increase blood pressure. Unlike our ancestors, it is very unlikely that the stress we experience will lead either to fight or flight (both of which, incidentally, would use up calories and help keep one fit). Instead the hormones will affect our blood pressure and if the stress is frequent or continuous, as is often the case in modern life, then this can lead to long-term problems with high blood pressure – especially in the context of an unhealthy lifestyle with little exercise. So, if you recognise that you are under stress, please do take time to see what you might be able to do to reduce the stress in your life. Some aspects of this are described in more detail in chapter 20.

Stress is also often associated with drinking too much alcohol. Drinking in excess of the standard guidelines (14 units per week) is associated with a number of health problems, including a rise in blood pressure. So, if you drink more than this – and beware, many of us underestimate the amount of alcohol we drink – then it is likely to be contributing to high blood pressure, and I would recommend considering how you might cut down. I know of many people who have managed to do this quite successfully, by adopting some ground rules for drinking. Examples include: not drinking alcohol alone, not drinking at home, not having beer in the house and having two or three days each week when you will not drink alcohol. The important thing is that whatever you decide to do has to be realistic, something that you can keep up – and that is not too drastic. Having said that, I know of some people who decide to stop drinking alcohol completely – and succeed.

The third factor which increases blood pressure is salt. A higher salt level leads to more water remaining in the circulation, which if excessive, can lead to high blood pressure. Now given that we are largely made up of salty water (or saline), then it is clear that we need some salt in our diet. Indeed, people with too little salt can experience dizziness and fainting due to their blood pressure being too low. Very low salt concentrations in the blood can cause more severe problems, including brain damage. But our modern diet includes too much salt. And this is made worse in people with too much insulin, as insulin itself helps the body retain salt, exacerbating the problem. Here again, reducing your carbohydrate intake so that you need less insulin will help reduce excessive salt retention.

If your blood pressure is high, then reducing the salt in your diet can make a big difference. The first step is to try and avoid adding salt to your food at the table. Pepper or other spices can add taste with no effect on your blood pressure. Then you may consider reducing the amount of salt you add during cooking. Obviously, salt is important to enhance flavour, but not so much that you can actually taste the saltiness. However, the biggest challenge in reducing salt is knowing which foods contain it – and you may be surprised. Just about any processed savoury food (and many sweet foods) will likely have added salt. And this includes not only highly processed foods, which you may perceive to be unhealthy such as ready-made meals, but also more traditional foods such as bread, bacon and cheese. Sweet foods such as breakfast cereals may also contain salt. One reason salt is used is to add flavour to lower quality ingredients – you may find, therefore, that cheaper processed foods have a higher salt content than more expensive ones. In the UK we are fortunate in that many companies have voluntarily reduced the salt content of their foods, and now have lower salt concentrations than their counterparts in other parts of the world. If you follow the suggestions in this book, then you will likely eat more fresh foods and less processed food, and this will help reduce your intake of salt as well as of sugar and fat.

We have already discussed how increasing your physical activity can help you lose weight and improve your diabetes control. The same changes you decide to make in order to increase your activity level will, over time, also contribute to reducing your blood pressure. If you are significantly overweight, then reducing your body weight will certainly help reduce your blood pressure.

It may be, especially if you have had diabetes for some time, that despite making changes to your lifestyle and your diet, that your blood pressure is still too high. In this situation, you might need to take medication to reduce your blood pressure. There are several types of tablets for high blood pressure and those most commonly used for people with diabetes include groups of drugs called ACE inhibitors or ARBs. Examples of these are shown in the table below. Both of these have additional actions in protecting the kidney from the effects of diabetes and are relatively free from side-effects. In fact, the most common side-effect from ACE inhibitors is that they can cause a troublesome, dry cough. If that happens, then switching to an ARB will usually help resolve the problem. It is important that kidney function is checked periodically if on treatment with an ACE inhibitor or ARB. They should also be stopped during acute illness of dehydration (e.g. diarrhoea and vomiting). Other common blood pressure tables include mild diuretics (water tablets), calcium-channel blockers, alpha-blockers and beta-blockers. It is not uncommon that a combination of three or more different blood pressure drugs are required to achieve good blood pressure control.

Drugs used to treat high blood pressure.

Class of drug	Examples	Possible side-effects
ACE inhibitor	Ramipril Perindopril Lisinopril	Cough May worsen kidney function
ARB	Candesartan Irbesartan Losartan	May worsen kidney function
Thiazide diuretic	Bendroflumethazide chlorthalidone	Low sodium level

Class of drug	Examples	Possible side-effects
Calcium channel blocker	Amlodipine Felodipine nifedipine	Ankle swelling
Alpha blocker	Doxasozin	Ankle swelling Dizziness on standing
Beta blocker	Bisoprolol Carvedilol Atenolol	Slow pulse

Some people may experience different side-effects from certain blood pressure tablets. For example, I have known people feel 'spaced out' on a particular tablet, or experience vomiting. If this happens, then it is important to identify which tablet is causing it, and find another one which does not cause the problem. One side-effect, which is quite common, is that of erectile dysfunction which, as we discussed earlier, can also result from the effects of diabetes. Why, therefore, should a tablet designed to protect your health make it more difficult to get an erection? The answer lies in the fact that an erection arises as a result of blood spaces in the penis filling up with blood. This requires a good blood flow to be delivered by the arteries supplying the penis. People with high blood pressure are likely to have a degree of narrowing of the arteries (vascular disease, as discussed in chapter 18), which will cause reduced blood flow. Taking a tablet which reduces the blood pressure in the whole circulation, is likely to reduce the blood flow to the penis even more, hence making it more difficult to get an erection. This is why this problem can occur with a variety of different blood pressure medications. Fortunately, tablets such as Viagra, which opens the blood spaces in the penis to increase the flow of blood into them, can help in this situation.

Earlier, I mentioned how useful it is to be able to monitor your blood pressure at home, to ensure that it is under good control.

Measuring your blood pressure at home is even more useful if you are on medication. Indeed, I often encourage people to measure their own blood pressure to determine what dose of medication they need. If their blood pressure is still too high after a week on a particular dose, I would provide advice on increasing the dose without the need to consult me or a GP. Similarly, if home blood pressure measurements become too low, then with the correct advice, people can become empowered to reduce their medication. If you are on medication for your blood pressure, I would strongly advise you to purchase a monitor so you can keep a check on it yourself. My general advice is to check it once a week, and if it is still too high, to seek advice on how to adjust the medication. You can then take responsibility for ensuring your treatment is keeping your blood pressure where it should be.

To summarise, people with diabetes have a tendency to high blood pressure. High blood pressure accelerates some of the complications of diabetes. It is therefore very important that you keep your blood pressure as normal as possible, that is below 135/85. Changing your lifestyle to get more active, to reduce the salt in your diet and to lose weight will all help. Taking medication is often also necessary, and it is very helpful to monitor your blood pressure yourself, to ensure that the treatment is doing what it should be. Finally, you should be aware of the possible side-effects of switching to a different treatment.

If your blood pressure is normal, it is really important that it is checked at least once a year, and if it rises above 135/85 that you seek advice on whether treatment is required. You cannot tell if your blood pressure is high – the only way of knowing is to have it checked.

The other important risk factor for large vessel disease, which causes so many problems, is high cholesterol. Now, the body needs cholesterol for many functions. Cell membranes, which control what enters into the cells of the body, are largely made of cholesterol.

Vitamin D, essential for healthy bones, and many hormones are also made from cholesterol. However, our modern lifestyles mean that too many of us have too much cholesterol in our bloodstream and this can increase the risk of the narrowing of the arteries, which can lead to heart attacks, strokes and gangrene.

There are several types of cholesterol which have different actions. LDL-cholesterol is made in the liver; its role is to transport fats around the body. Too much LDL-cholesterol is associated with vascular disease. HDL-cholesterol, on the other hand, is good for you, as its role is to transport fats from the bloodstream and back to the liver. As a rule, it is recommended that your cholesterol levels should be as follows:

Total cholesterol less than 5mmol/l (200mg/dl)
LDL cholesterol less than 3mmol/l (120mg/dl)
HDL cholesterol MORE than 1mmol/l (40mg/dl)

People who already have evidence of large vessel disease, or who are at high risk of it, are advised to achieve lower targets. Now, some people have a high total cholesterol, but this is because there is a high level of healthy HDL. For this reason, it is often easiest to look just at the LDL cholesterol when deciding if you need to make any changes. As with high blood pressure, there are no symptoms associated with having a high cholesterol level, and so it is important to have a blood test done once every year to check your cholesterol level.

If your cholesterol levels are higher than they should be, then it is important that you know what you can do, to reduce them. As with high blood pressure, the first things to consider are whether there are any changes you can make to your lifestyle. And the good news is that exactly the same changes which help reduce your blood pressure also help reduce your cholesterol level. So, increasing your activity level, eating a healthy diet, and losing weight will all help. And beware of being taken in by low-fat foods. While there may seem to be a certain logic that eating less fat will reduce your cholesterol level, remember that insulin is the main fat-producing hormone, and that reducing your carbohydrate intake will help reduce the amount of insulin you need, as well as help improve your diabetes control. Remember also that healthy people on a ketogenic diet can also have quite raised cholesterol levels, as described in chapter 12.

Some people will be advised to take medication to reduce their cholesterol levels. The most common type of medication for high cholesterol levels nowadays is a class of drug called statins (such as simvastatin or atorvastatin). Statins all work in a similar way, by reducing the amount of cholesterol released from the liver into the bloodstream. They are undoubtedly effective in reducing cholesterol and are generally well-tolerated, and only need to be taken once a day. However, they can cause side-effects, particularly if used at higher doses. The commonest side-effects are muscle aches and pains, which can sometimes be associated with a potentially serious inflammation of the muscles known as myositis. As statins have become more widely used, a number of other side-effects have been reported, ranging from headaches to difficulty sleeping, joint pains and poor concentration. If you feel that you have experienced a new symptom since taking a statin, my advice would be to stop the statin for a few weeks. Generally, if the symptom is related to the statin, it will soon end after stopping it. It may be that you will manage better with a lower dose of the statin, or with a different statin. Occasionally alternative types of medication may be required.

Statins are of benefit for those who have had a vascular event, such as a heart attack, or who are at high risk of one. The UK NICE guidelines also recommend that everyone with type 1 diabetes over the age of 40 or who has had the condition for over ten years should be offered treatment with a statin, even if they are otherwise very healthy. Some of my patients have questioned this advice, as the absolute benefit of taking a statin for any individual in this situation is actually quite small. The NICE guidelines do emphasise that the decision to take a statin should be based on a discussion between the person with diabetes and their doctor, and should take the individual's preferences into account. Thus, if it has been suggested that you take a statin, be reassured that at the end of the day, it is your choice as to whether you do. You may also be encouraged by evidence that suggests that adopting a Mediterranean type of diet (characterised by a high intake of fresh vegetables, nuts and of healthy fats such as those in olive oil and oily fish) is at least as effective in reducing the risk of vascular disease as taking a statin.[67]

To summarise the key messages about cholesterol: have a blood test to get it checked every year, know what your level is and, if it is high, seek advice about how you can reduce it. Meanwhile, adopting lifestyle changes recommended in this book will help you on your way.

Both high blood pressure and high cholesterol contribute to many of the complications of diabetes. Keeping them under good control will help reduce the risk of complications.

20

DEALING WITH DIABETES-RELATED DISTRESS

From the preceding chapters, you will have learnt how having type
1 diabetes can affect many aspects of daily living – both as a result
of the disease itself or health problems related to your diabetes, or
because you must undertake a series of lifestyle changes needed
to manage your diabetes. You will also have learnt how everyday
activities can affect type 1 diabetes, especially concerning food intake
and activity levels. And we have discussed how illness can also affect
diabetes. In short: type 1 diabetes can affect many aspects of everyday
life, and many aspects of everyday life can affect type 1 diabetes. It
is little wonder, therefore, that at times having type 1 diabetes can
cause stress, anxiety and even depression. In addition, a person with
diabetes may have psychological issues that are unrelated to their
diabetes. Regardless of its cause, stress, anxiety or depression can all
impact on a person's ability to manage their diabetes.

Over the years, I have seen a number of people with type 1 diabetes who have experienced devastating health problems, often at young age, as a result of poor control of their diabetes. In too many cases, the reasons for this were, at least in part, psychological. I can think of individuals who ran very high glucose levels as they had an overwhelming fear of a really bad hypo. Usually this was in turn as a result of a bad experience with a hypo, sometimes many years ago. The hypo may have occurred when they were a child, when they were on (by today's standards) rather primitive insulin or may even have been before they had access to home blood testing. There may be plenty of logical reasons why such a devastating hypo would now be much less likely to happen. Despite this, the emotional reaction has dictated how they manage their diabetes many years later, with sometimes catastrophic results.

Others experience negative reactions to doing blood glucose checks on themselves. Such negative reactions could result for example from painful early experiences of being restrained as a small child so a blood test could be done, or from fear of the result of the test, perhaps associated with a degree of helplessness about what to do about the result if it shows a very high glucose level.

Others might have developed a coping mechanism to the diagnosis of type 1 diabetes by going into denial about it. I recall one young lady who ignored her diabetes throughout her teens and early twenties until she was about to get married, to the extent that until then her husband was unaware about the importance of managing diabetes well in order to stay healthy in the future. You can imagine the strain that such issues could place on a relationship between a newly-married couple.

Still others may have experienced abuse in early life, possibly even before they developed type 1 diabetes. As a result, they were consumed with feelings of shame and low self-worth. Sometimes that translates into a feeling that they are somehow not worthy of the effort required to keep their diabetes under control.

Whatever the issue, and there are many more possible examples I could cite, having a negative emotional or psychological reaction to any aspect of diabetes (or anything else) could contribute to you being unable to achieve stable control of your diabetes. And that of course will have a direct impact on your physical health, if not in the short term, then certainly in the long term.

By contrast, if you do not have diabetes, and you have a psychological reaction to an unpleasant experience in the past, that may affect your mood at times. It may also affect certain behaviours, but unless it leads to excessive drinking, or massive overeating, it is unlikely to have an imminent and direct impact on your physical health.

As a result of seeing people struggle with these issues, I became convinced very early on in my career of the need for everyone with type 1 diabetes to have access to expert psychological support. To many in my profession, this is a nice-to-have 'optional extra'. To me it is essential as, for the reasons I have explained, with type 1 diabetes in the mix, poor psychological health can directly lead to poor physical health. Note I say *expert* psychological support is needed. By that, I mean support from a health professional who is an expert in psychological assessment and treatment and also an expert in type 1 diabetes. They need to understand the realities, the complexities and the challenges of living with diabetes, how these impact psychological health and what can be done to alleviate them. All too often in my experience, experts in psychology did not also have expertise in diabetes, and were therefore unable to help, except at a superficial level. Imagine my delight then, soon after I arrived at Bournemouth, when I referred a young person to the local psychology service. By then I was used to getting the usual rather bland letter explaining the issues but then saying 'of course they have diabetes so the options for helping them are limited' (I paraphrase). But this time, I got a letter in which the psychologist expressed her interest in the case, and invited me to send more patients to her, if required.

That psychologist was Clare Shaban, and that letter was all I needed to get straight back to her and to invite her to join with me in helping set up a psychological service for people with diabetes in Bournemouth. That was in 1996 and at the time she had been designated to provide a psychological service for a half-day each week not just to my department, but to the whole hospital where I worked. At that time, any patients I referred to her had to travel to see her at the psychiatric hospital where she was based, and so the first thing I did was to invite her to see patients within our department. This was for two reasons. Firstly, I wanted to send a signal to those people who would need her help that this was part of the treatment for their diabetes, available from within our department and not requiring a separate visit to a psychiatric hospital. Secondly, and more mischievously, I wanted her to spend as much of her allocated half-day on people with diabetes, although she could of course see people with other conditions as required.

It soon became apparent that half a day a week was nowhere near enough time to meet the needs of our population with diabetes. I therefore set out to get some funding for her to do a research project that I hoped would demonstrate the need for the service. The project aimed to assess the psychological health of everyone with type 1 diabetes who came into our department'. At the same time, we started to offer psychological assessment as part of the care for everyone newly diagnosed with type 1 diabetes, initially as a separate consultation, but since 2004 as part of the Living with Diabetes programme.

The results of the early research confirmed that there was some evidence of more severe depression, particularly in men with type

1 diabetes. The more significant problem, however, was of more severe anxiety, particularly in women.[68] Further analysis showed that higher anxiety was associated with higher HbA1c levels and that it was generally as a result of diabetes-specific distress.[69]

The term 'diabetes distress' has been introduced to describe the emotional and psychological burden experienced by people with diabetes. As diabetes distress is associated with higher HbA1c levels,[70] and increased risk of diabetes-related complications, there is growing recognition that it needs to be taken more seriously.

The DAWN2 study was a large study that was undertaken in seventeen countries around the world in 2011.[71] It looked specifically at the psychological, educational and emotional needs of people with diabetes and came up with some very interesting results. Nearly half of all people with diabetes reported high levels of diabetes distress and one in seven people had such low emotional wellbeing that they were likely to be suffering from depression. The study also found that diabetes had a negative impact on family and other relationships, on leisure activities, work and finances. So, what causes diabetes distress?

Diabetes distress is likely to result from a number of factors that affect people with the disease. These include how well they accept the diagnosis of diabetes, how they adjust to the lifestyle changes required to control it, and how they cope with complications if they arise. Even in the absence of long-term complications, just having high blood glucose levels can affect mood or the ability to concentrate, as well as cause unpleasant physical symptoms such as thirst, frequent urination, thrush and erectile dysfunction. These readily explain how having diabetes can affect relationships, family life and employment. It is also easy to imagine how someone, burdened by these problems, might find it more difficult to focus on the blood tests, insulin injections and attention to diet that are needed to control type 1 diabetes.

Indeed, diabetes distress has been shown to be associated with lower levels of physical activity, poor diet and reduced adherence to prescribed treatments. This in turn explains why diabetes distress is associated with worse control of diabetes, which in turn increases the risk of complications, which in themselves will likely further exacerbate diabetes distress – creating a vicious circle as shown in the figure.

having diabetes

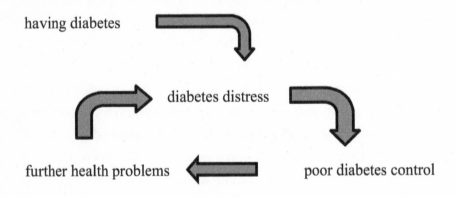

diabetes distress

further health problems   poor diabetes control

As we discussed in chapter 8, the way people are managed when they are first diagnosed with diabetes creates a significant mental impression; and it's something that can stay with them for many years. Not only does it impact on a person's diabetes control and physical health, but also on his or her psychological health. For many people being diagnosed with diabetes comes as a nasty shock – and may be associated with a number of different emotions:

Fear: if they know someone who has suffered from diabetes in the past, especially if that individual had a bad time with it.

Resentment: if they resent their loss of health and the consequent freedom to eat and do whatever they want.

Isolation: if they happen to be the only one amongst family and/or friends with diabetes.

Guilt: if they think that diabetes results from their own actions, such as gaining too much weight (more common in people with type 2 diabetes).

Confusion: if they have been given inappropriate advice on what they should or should not eat, perhaps from a well-meaning relative.

Helplessness: if they believe their diabetes will gradually get worse, regardless of what they do.

Some of these powerful emotions are the product of the thoughts, feelings and worries that naturally emerge within the person who is newly diagnosed, but others arise from the things that are communicated by people around them, who may previously have had second-hand experiences of other people's diabetes. Regardless of their origin, I believe it is important that everyone at diagnosis of diabetes has an opportunity to express their feelings, and to receive high quality education about how they can best manage their diabetes going forward. Getting the right information at the beginning can help correct any misinformation that may lead to negative emotions.

Another source of diabetes distress arises from the conventional approach to diet in type 1 diabetes. As previously discussed, there is a widely-held belief amongst many health professionals that if you have type 1 diabetes, you can eat whatever you like, as long as you take the right amount of insulin. I used to believe that myself. This, coupled with the belief that it is healthy to eat plenty of carbohydrates, risked setting people up to failure. A carbohydrate-rich diet, despite containing 'healthy' carbohydrates, risks causing high blood glucose levels, and further causing confusion and despondency in someone who believes they are doing 'the right thing'. I would therefore anticipate that a more emphatic focus on using diet to help keep glucose levels down, coupled with a simple explanation about which foods will do this, will help people feel they are in control of their condition. And will in turn reduce feelings of helplessness and of anxiety.

The DAWN2 study showed that people who received education about their diabetes felt better equipped to manage their diabetes, were more actively involved in their care, received more support and reported better wellbeing. It is recognised that access to good quality information about diabetes, as well as self-management education, can help reduce anxiety related to diabetes. Modern education programmes place an emphasis not just on how to manage diabetes, but also in developing goal-setting, problem-solving and coping skills so that when things go wrong, as occasionally they will, the individual is well-equipped to deal with them. This highlights the importance of self-management education in helping reduce diabetes distress.

The long-term complications of diabetes are an obvious source of diabetes distress. Experiencing visual loss, a foot ulcer or erectile dysfunction will inevitably be a cause of huge anxiety. When complications arise, it is right that the immediate priority is given to the medical treatments that will help manage the complication. However, it is important that the person with diabetes, as well as his or her health care team, recognise the emotional effects complications may have on their mental well-being, and are provided with both support and appropriate treatment for any mental distress. If you are in this situation, and you feel you have not been offered appropriate support, please discuss it with someone in your diabetes team.

Not all health professionals are aware of the concept of diabetes distress, and it can sometimes be confused with depression. However, depression is different. With depression, people often have negative thoughts about themselves and a sense of hopelessness about the future. Diabetes distress, on the other hand, is associated with thoughts and feelings specifically about diabetes. While these could be negative and be associated with a sense of hopelessness about the future, they can be helped by addressing the diabetes-related issues that led to them, whether it be high glucose levels, hypos or a specific symptom, for example.

Clare Shaban provides the following tips for avoiding diabetes distress. These, and other information about the psychological aspects of having diabetes, can be found in the Lifewise section of the BERTIEonline website:

- Give yourself permission to feel 'negative' emotions like frustration and anger towards diabetes – they are a healthy response to its demands.
- Look after yourself when you are going through a stressful life event. Diabetes control may need to be given less priority for a time, until life has returned to 'normal'. Consider the minimum you need to do to care for your health.
- Strive for balance in your life – your diabetes health is important, but so are your social relationships, rest and play. Try to give time to each.
- Aim for realistic goals rather than perfectionistic standards. Be kind to yourself.
- Think of one self-care task you are avoiding which you could do today, and congratulate or reward yourself for doing it.
- Talk to someone involved in your diabetes care about the way you are feeling about your diabetes.
- It can help to talk about your experiences of diabetes to others who understand. Internet forums are a good way to do this.

In more recent years in Bournemouth we used the Problem Areas in Diabetes (PAID) Scale to assess diabetes distress in different groups of people with type 1 diabetes, and to track changes in relation to different interventions (such as following diagnosis, attending a BERTIE course or starting on an insulin pump). We have found that each of these is associated with often dramatic improvements in diabetes distress and this does seem to support the theory that if individuals can be supported in achieving stable management of their diabetes, then many of the signs of anxiety do begin to lessen. As the aim of this book is to provide you with the tools to manage your diabetes, my hope is that any diabetes distress you may have experienced will reduce with time once you learn how you can take control of, and live more normally with, your diabetes. However, if you have more deep-seated issues that are affecting your ability to achieve control of your diabetes, as with the examples I mentioned at the start of this chapter, then you may need additional support. Therefore, if you continue to experience anxiety or low-mood relating to your diabetes, or to another problem, please seek help.

Depression does occur in people with diabetes and is often associated with low motivation and also with low self-worth. These make it more difficult to make changes to diet or to keep to a demanding treatment regimen. Therefore, it is likely that if you are depressed you will find it far more challenging to make the changes necessary to control your diabetes; the depression may need to be treated first.

The National Institute for Health and Clinical Excellence (NICE) states that healthcare professionals working in diabetes teams should be alert to the development or presence of depression or anxiety, especially in people who find it difficult to manage their diabetes. They should also be able to detect and manage non-severe psychological disorders, and have access to more specialist psychological services for the more complex problems. Unfortunately, specialist psychological provision is not routine in many diabetes centres in the UK. However, this must not put you off from seeking treatment if you need it.

In summary, diabetes distress is a very common problem, arising from different aspects of having diabetes. It can result in negative emotions, anxiety and low-mood, which make it difficult to manage diabetes. Ensuring you are properly educated in how to manage your diabetes and knowing how to deal with setbacks when they arise can all help improve diabetes distress – although more severe symptoms may require psychological or medical treatments.

21

TOWARDS A CURE FOR TYPE 1 DIABETES

At the beginning, I talked about the need that we all have for hope. As you read the subsequent chapters, it would be understandable if you felt rather devoid of hope at times. However, I firmly believe there are more grounds for hope in type 1 diabetes than at any time in my career. While a cure in the true sense may seem a long way off, there are a number of exciting developments which suggest it will happen. And others that in the meantime will transform the management of type 1 diabetes. In this chapter, I will present the state of play in 2018.

THE ARTIFICIAL PANCREAS

Although not strictly speaking a cure, to many people the idea of an artificial pancreas would come very close to a cure. Earlier we discussed insulin pumps and continuous glucose monitors, which can both offer distinct benefits to users. What is really exciting is the possibility of linking these two systems together to form what is known as a closed-loop system, or artificial pancreas.

The first step in the evolution of the artificial pancreas has been the development of sensor-augmented pumps (SAPs) as described in chapter 13. These suspend insulin delivery if the sensor measures hypoglycaemia. More advanced versions suspend insulin delivery, based on a prediction that a hypo will occur, if no action is taken. The logical next step is for the system to respond to high glucose measurements by increasing the insulin infusion. This is relatively easy (actually it's very complicated) during the night, or during periods when a person is inactive and not eating; it becomes much more complex when physical activity levels and food intake have to be taken into consideration. In other words, the closed loop system can only react to the glucose levels that it measures, it cannot know, for example that today you are going to eat a pizza or go for a 10km run. You need to tell it.

Such hybrid closed loop systems, where the mealtime insulin doses are determined by the user (using a bolus advisor for example), have been under development in recent years. The initial studies were done under laboratory conditions, and showed that the systems were safe to use overnight. Subsequent studies were done on people using the system overnight at home, but with remote monitoring of glucose levels as a safety precaution. One such study lasted six weeks, and showed that time spent with hypoglycaemic blood glucose levels was reduced by half.[72] Subsequently, 'free living' studies in people using the overnight closed-loop system for up to two months confirmed their benefit and safety.[73] Finally, studies have been done for up to three months where people used the closed loop system during the day as well as at night.[74] These confirmed the safety and benefit of the closed-loop systems in improving glucose control and reducing hypoglycaemia, compared with standard pump therapy. In 2016, the first such system (Medtronic MiniMed 670G) was approved for use in the US.[75] It became available for use in 2017 in the US and there is as yet no news about its roll out in Europe or elsewhere. When it does become available in the UK, it will likely initially only be available on the NHS for people at high risk of hypoglycaemia. However, it is a very exciting development and I expect that it will become more widely available over the next ten years.

These systems can prevent hypoglycaemia by reducing insulin delivery rate. Meanwhile at the research level, so-called dual-loop systems that use not only insulin, but also glucagon, are under development. Glucagon is a hormone produced by the pancreas that, unlike insulin, increases glucose levels. In theory, using glucagon will enable glucose levels to be increased more effectively than using insulin alone. A number of studies have shown such systems to be safe and reliable, although one system that was 'fully closed-loop', that is without manual mealtime boluses, was associated with more hypoglycaemia than standard pump therapy during a two-day study period.[76] There are also a number of technical challenges, as to date glucagon in liquid form has a short shelf-life.

ISLET CELL TRANSPLANTATION

As we learnt in chapter 2, insulin is produced by beta cells located in clumps or 'islets' of cells found in the pancreas. Islet cell transplantation describes the procedure in which islets from a deceased person are transplanted into a person with type 1 diabetes. It is a very complex process that requires a pancreas from two deceased persons. The pancreases are then digested by enzymes to release the islets. The islets are then 'purified' to ensure they are completely separated from the other pancreatic tissue, and then injected into a portal vein in the liver that receives blood containing glucose absorbed from the gut. The transplanted islets then attach to blood vessels in the liver, and within a few weeks begin producing insulin in response to the amount of glucose in the vessels. This process has developed since early research in the 1960s. By the 1990s, early recipients saw success with 'reversal' of their type 1 diabetes, meaning they no longer need to inject insulin. However, these were in the minority; in up to 90 per cent of cases, individuals still required insulin, indicating that the transplanted islets were functioning only poorly or not at all. Now, as with all transplantation procedures, recipients have to take immunosuppressant medications in order to prevent their immune system from rejecting the islets. Up until the 1990s these included steroids. One of the important effects of steroids is to increase blood glucose levels and it was thought that this might have played a role in limiting the effectiveness of the transplanted islets.

In 2000, there was much excitement in the diabetes community. Dr James Shapiro from Edmonton in Canada had developed a protocol for islet transplantation that did not require steroids as part of the immunosuppression treatment.[77] The initial results were very encouraging, and seven people who received islet transplants now had normal glucose levels. I remember hearing Dr Shapiro give a lecture at a conference at the time. It was one of those moments when you feel that history was being made, as here was, apparently, a cure for type 1 diabetes. He, himself, though, acknowledged that it was not going to be a universal cure, as it required at least two pancreases for each transplant (bear in mind that one dead person can donate a kidney each to two separate individuals); rather the techniques he had developed could be adapted to use stem cells that have been 'grown' to produce insulin.

Nevertheless, there was much hope that the procedure would offer a ray of hope to some people with diabetes, and Diabetes UK provided funding to set up islet cell transplantation in the UK. Quite quickly, however, it became apparent that the early hope was not to be fulfilled. Many people needed to start insulin within a year of their transplant, some were never able to stop insulin, and by five years, 90 per cent needed some insulin. However, those that had experienced significant problems with hypoglycaemia before the transplant found that their diabetes was much easier to control afterwards. It quickly became seen as a treatment for people with disabling hypoglycaemia, rather than a 'cure' for type 1 diabetes.

However, by then, insulin pump technology and new insulin analogues were providing alternative and less invasive means of achieving the same goal, but without the need for potentially dangerous immunosuppressant therapy. Personally, therefore, I did not feel that islet cell transplantation in its current form was a necessary option for most people with type 1 diabetes. Although a few of my patients explored islet cell transplantation and some visited the regional transplant centre, none of them actually decided to proceed with the procedure. It does remain an option for people who still experience disabling hypoglycaemia, despite insulin pump therapy and continued glucose monitoring. Meanwhile, further research in underway to improve the success of islet cell transplantation. One approach is to protect the cells in capsules that allow nutrients to reach the cells but protect them from attack by immune cells.

USING STEM CELLS TO PRODUCE INSULIN

The tissues in the body are all made up of individual units called cells. The body has many types of different cells that perform very different functions. Think of a muscle cell in the heart that changes shape to cause the heart to contract, or of a gut cell that absorbs digested food from the gut into the bloodstream, or of a nerve cell that carries pain sensation from the tip of your toe to the spinal cord. Then think of an islet cell, whose job is to monitor the level of glucose in the tissues and produce exactly the right amount of insulin. All very, very different in their shape and what they can do. Yet they all started out as identical, primitive stem cells. Such cells have been the focus of research into treatments for a number of different conditions in recent years, with some success.

The most primitive stem cells come from embryos, and much early work used embryonic stem cells. The advantage of these is that they can be programmed to develop into any type of cell and that there is a ready supply. Stem cells can be obtained from embryos created for use in in-vitro fertilisation (IVF) treatment. Often, not all embryos are required or suitable and would otherwise be destroyed. Stem cells from these embryos can be propagated indefinitely for research. However, their use raises ethical questions, to the extent that in 2001 President George W Bush restricted even the use of these embryos for research, as it required 'the destruction of human life'. Nevertheless, it was in the US that in 2014 Dr Doug Melton announced that his team at Harvard University was successful in producing large quantities of insulin-producing cells from embryonic stem cells,[78] the crucial first step necessary for stem cell therapy to be a possibility for the cure of type 1 diabetes. A team led by Dr Timothy Kieffer at the University of British Columbia in Canada achieved the same feat at almost exactly the same time.[79] The cells developed are being used in further research to discover the best way to make that possibility a reality.

Stem cells are also present in a number of tissues in adults. They are used as part of the body's continuous repair process. Such cells are less flexible than embryonic stem cells, as they are already partly programmed to develop into certain cell types. Nevertheless, they can still be used to develop potential treatments for specific conditions, related to their function. For example, bone marrow transplants are a form of stem cell therapy, where stem cells in bone marrow are used as a treatment for some forms of leukaemia. There is evidence that some stem cells are present in the pancreas; although these are rare, they could potentially be programmed as insulin-producing cells.

It has also been shown that adult stem cells can be reprogrammed from their original function, and even that mature cells can be reprogrammed to become stem cells. One example of the use of stem cell therapy that will be of interest to many men with type 1 diabetes, is research undertaken in Denmark, and reported in 2017. Fat cells were removed from the abdomen, reprogrammed and injected into the penis, where they develop into nerve cells, muscle cells and endothelial cells (that line blood vessels).[80] This proved an effective treatment for erectile dysfunction in an initial trial and further research in ongoing.

It will be some years before stem cell therapy becomes a viable option for the treatment of type 1 diabetes, but when it does, I believe it will provide the nearest to a cure of all the developments discussed in this chapter.

WHOLE PANCREAS TRANSPLANTATION

The nearest currently-available procedure to a cure for type 1 diabetes is a whole-pancreas transplant. Unlike an islet cell transplant, this involves a major operation to transplant a whole pancreas into the abdomen. Also unlike an islet cell transplant, however, it offers a much higher chance of success. So, both the risks and the benefits are greater. A whole pancreas transplant can be done as a stand-alone procedure, for much the same reasons as an islet cell transplant. Given my previous comments about how insulin pump and CGM technology can now overcome many of the problems that were previously experienced with hypos, it stands that there must be compelling reasons to recommend a whole pancreas transplant. Indeed, the few people who I referred for a pancreas transplant had specific issues which made insulin treatment, even with a pump, very difficult. In most cases it was successful in meaning the person no longer needed insulin treatment.

A whole pancreas transplant is transformational when it is performed at the same time as a kidney transplant. By definition, therefore, these are performed in individuals who had kidney failure, usually also with many other complications because of their diabetes. At the time of their transplant, they are either already on kidney dialysis or are very near to needing it. They are usually very ill, on many medications and frequently requiring admission to hospital. It is not exaggerating to say that some of my patients who underwent a pancreas and kidney transplant were close to death. With his permission, I will describe the case of one young man whose life was completely transformed by receiving a new kidney and pancreas.

He developed type 1 diabetes as a young child and I first got to know him when he was about 30 years old. By then he had very high blood pressure that was difficult to control. He had diabetic retinopathy and had required laser treatment in the past. He had neuropathy that affected his gut, causing nausea and vomiting, and loss of sensation in his feet. He also had retrograde ejaculation. His blood pressure was very difficult to control, and required a combination of medications that at times made him feel very light-headed and exacerbated his nausea and vomiting. His blood glucose was unstable, and he told me how in his younger years, he experienced some really bad hypos. So much so, that he was sometimes fearful of going to bed, as he never knew whether he would have a hypo in the night, whether he would wake up in hospital, or whether he would wake up at all. Such bad experiences understandably led him to want to keep his blood glucose higher than ideal, but tragically that contributed to his worsening complications later on.

A couple of years after I first met him, his kidneys began to fail. As they did, he became more and more unwell, and his symptoms worsened. He had several admissions to hospital with dehydration due to vomiting, high glucose levels and high blood pressure. He was on the verge of giving up hope and stopping taking his treatments. He was no longer able to work. He was assessed for a kidney and pancreas transplant, passed the various assessments and was put on the list for surgery. It then came to the point where he would soon need dialysis to keep him alive. In preparation for this, he had a fistula created in his arm. This is a connection between an artery and a vein that is used to access the blood supply during dialysis. It is usually a routine procedure, but unfortunately in his case it led to quite severe damage to one of the main nerves in his arm that became painful and weak as a result.

Then in December 2006, at the age of 35, he received a call from the regional transplant centre. A pancreas and kidney were available that were a good match for him. He underwent surgery that lasted about eight hours. During the operation, the new kidney was inserted into the lower left part of his abdomen, and connected to the renal blood vessels and to the bladder. The new pancreas was inserted into the right part of his abdomen and connected to blood vessels into which insulin would be secreted. As the whole pancreas is transplanted, then it also produces digestive enzymes that are secreted into the gut. This part of the pancreas was therefore connected to his gut. His own pancreas and kidneys were left in place.

The surgery was a success. Within hours both his new pancreas and his new kidney were working normally. By the time he left hospital he was no longer on insulin, and he has remained off insulin and free from diabetes ever since. Within days, he reported that his legs began to feel normal again, for the first time for years. Over the next few weeks, many of his medications were discontinued, including several for blood pressure and nausea. Gradually the strength in his arm returned, completely to normal. He was able to go back to work and for the first time in his adult life experienced good health. So much so that he and his wife were able to contemplate starting a family. Three years following his transplant, he became the proud father of twins. Now, over ten years since his transplant, he is free from all traces of his diabetes. Even the eye clinic has discharged him as his eyes show no signs of active retinopathy. Of course, he still must take his antirejection immunosuppressive medications, and attend a review once a year to check all is well. However, many of the long-term complications of diabetes that we used to believe were irreversible had reversed. His kidney failure could only be reversed with a new kidney, however, the new pancreas ensured his glucose levels were normal and that allowed his nerves, stomach and eyes to repair themselves. The new pancreas also protected the new kidney from further damage from high glucose levels.

I have seen a number of people who have similar success stories following a pancreas and kidney transplant, but none quite as dramatic as this one. There were also some less successful outcomes. Overall, however, the procedure is very successful and a recent analysis of UK cases has shown that one year after the operation, 97 per cent of patients are alive with 85 per cent of pancreases working normally.[81]

IMMUNE THERAPY AND REVERSAL OF TYPE 1 DIABETES

The final type of 'cure' for type 1 diabetes is immune therapy directed at stopping the body's immune system from attacking the insulin-producing beta cells. It is thought that an effective treatment given soon after the onset of type 1 diabetes could halt the immune attack and enable insulin production to continue, before it is permanently affected, that is, during the honeymoon period. Such a treatment would also be important to help increase the survival of treatments such as islet cell transplants. A range of different therapies are currently undergoing evaluation to identify one or more that will be effective.

There has been a lot of excitement in recent years at the discovery that the underlying metabolic abnormalities in type 2 diabetes can be reversed by lifestyle change. Until then, it was believed that once you got it, you would have type 2 diabetes for life, and almost whatever you did, it was an inexorably progressive condition. So far, it is still generally accepted that type 1 diabetes cannot be reversed. While I think this is a safe assumption with our current knowledge, there are some intriguing developments at research level that are beginning to question this assumption.

Studies have looked at the potential role of the BCG vaccine (as used for tuberculosis) in attacking the immune cells that attack the beta cells. Early studies showed there was some return of insulin secretion, leading to the intriguing prospect that type 1 diabetes could one day be reversed.[82] More recently, an article was published that described an experiment in which mice with type 1 diabetes were subject to a fasting-mimicking diet (essentially a low-calorie, low-carbohydrate, high-fat diet) for four days. This was associated with increased insulin secretion, thought to be due to reprogramming of the beta cells to produce insulin.[83] Now this doesn't prove that type 1 diabetes in humans could be reversed, but it does at least suggest that in the nearest mouse equivalent, the beta cells are still capable of producing insulin, if only we can identify the best way of helping them do so in the long term.

Finally, a group in Hungary recommend a paleo-ketogenic (low-carbohydrate, high animal fat) diet for type 1 diabetes. They believe that certain foods are associated with inflammation in the gut that leads to a 'leaky gut' that allows substances to enter the bloodstream. This triggers an immune response that in turn increases the risk for a number of autoimmune diseases, including type 1 diabetes. They have written a report of how a 19-year-old man with newly-diagnosed type 1 diabetes responded to such a diet. He was able to stop insulin and remain free from insulin for over six months.[84] In fact he remained off insulin until he resumed a normal diet after a year. Another individual was able to remain off insulin for two years; as soon as he returned to a normal diet he had to start insulin again. Now, six months is well within the timeframe for a honeymoon period in which a person may not require insulin; two years without insulin could still be feasible from a honeymoon period, although it is unusual not to require any insulin for that length of time. If it is proven that the need to take insulin is directly related to a change in diet, that would be very exciting indeed.

Some of these reports may sound a little far-fetched, and you may wonder why I have included them. I have done so, not to encourage people to adopt radical diets or to stop their insulin, but because I believe it is important to remain open-minded about the prospect of a cure for type 1 diabetes. I also firmly believe that hope is a very powerful motivator, even if the chance of such a cure seems very small; in my experience, hope is all too often in short supply in some diabetes departments.

If I reflect on the changes in the thirty years since I qualified as a doctor, it is not too fanciful to hope that there might be a cure. In the 1980s, surgeons regularly removed parts (or all) of a person's stomach as a treatment for stomach ulcers. At the time, they were thought to be due to stress. It is now known that a bacterial infection plays a large role, and antibiotics and medication that suppresses acid secretion mean that such operations are almost unheard of nowadays. Again, in the 1980s, AIDS was a terminal disease – often leading to death within months. Very few people develop AIDS anymore, even in the developing world, as HIV is controlled by low-cost medications that have turned it into a long-term condition, with which people can live for decades, not just for a few months. And closer to 'home', type 2 diabetes was thought to be related to genetics, and that once you had it, you had it for life. Just ten years ago, no one would have conceived that it could be reversed, yet now more and more people are doing just that, as we have learnt that it results from modern-day lifestyles.

So, a permanent cure for type 1 diabetes might be within our grasp based on our current understanding; it may yet happen, and depending on how old you are, within your lifetime. In the meantime, there are exciting new developments, unthinkable just ten years ago, that are already available to make the management of type 1 diabetes less burdensome, and others (such as the artificial pancreas) that will undoubtedly become more widely available over the next few years.

22

SETTING YOUR OWN GOALS, MAKING CHANGES AND STICKING TO THEM

If you have read this book from the beginning you will understand that almost everything you do affects your blood glucose control. You may already have a clear idea of the steps you can take to help stabilise and improve your glucose control, if that is needed. These can be broadly classified as:

1. changes to your diet and lifestyle to reduce your insulin requirements,
2. ensuring adequate blood glucose monitoring, and
3. where necessary, changes to your insulin dose or method of delivery.

Life is full of good intentions, many of which, if we're honest with ourselves, are never realised. Therefore, it is important that if you are about to make significant changes to your lifestyle or how you manage your diabetes, you set yourself realistic goals. It is equally important to be honest with yourself about how motivated you are to make these changes. Reading this book to this point probably hasn't been the most fun you've had. I sincerely hope, though, that most of it will have been interesting. But the fact that you have read the book through to this point suggests that you are at least sufficiently motivated to find out what you can do to take control of your diabetes.

If you have read through from the beginning, there is a good chance that you have already made some changes. If you have not yet done so, maybe you are actively considering making some changes in the next few weeks. If so, read on.

If you still do not feel ready to make changes in the next few weeks, I would suggest waiting until you do feel ready before committing to change. Here I want to point out that there is absolutely nothing wrong with not being ready to make changes. It is human nature that we all do the things we think are important for us right now. If, at the moment, you do not think it is important to make a change, then it's probably not worth trying; you will be setting yourself up to fail. That isn't the same thing as saying you do not understand how a change may be beneficial to your health; rather it is an acknowledgment that your current lifestyle, which perhaps includes a family or work situation that is consuming all of your energy, is more important to you right now.

We all know the merits of giving up cigarette smoking. Isn't it extraordinary how everyone knows how truly awful the habit is for his or her immediate and longer-term wellbeing, and yet people continue to smoke. The enjoyment people get from smoking (coupled with its addictive nature) proves to be more attractive than the processes of trying to give up something pleasurable now in order to derive health benefits in the future. The key is always – how ready you are to change? For you to assess this, it might be helpful to ask yourself two questions:

1. On a scale of zero (not at all important) to ten (extremely important), how important is it for me to make changes to take control of my diabetes?
2. On a scale of zero (not at all confident) to ten (extremely confident), how confident do I feel that I can make changes to take control of my diabetes?

In my clinical experience, most people to whom I put these questions give a high score (usually eight, nine or ten) to the first question. After all, they have chosen to come to see me to discuss their diabetes. However, the answers to the second question would usually vary quite a lot. If your answer to both questions is high (and you are being honest in your assessment!), then you are ready to change. However, if your answer to the second question is four or five (or less), then you should follow it up with some further questions:

3. What is the reason or reasons I chose to score so low to the second question?
4. What would need to happen for me to be able to give myself a higher score?

This may prompt you to focus on what are the barriers to you making the changes and addressing those barriers so that you are better able to make the changes.

If you are still with me I am assuming you feel that now is the time to have a go and to make some changes in your lifestyle or other aspects of managing your diabetes. And so, before going any further, I would like to return to the questions that were posed at the end of chapter 1. Even if you have answered them earlier, please spend some time now answering them as fully as you can. Write your answers down; it will be useful to refer to them in the future:

- What are your reasons for reading this book?
- What frustrates you most about having diabetes?
- How do you want things to be different?
- How will you know when you have achieved this?
- What is the main thing you would like to change after reading this book?

Your answer to the last question is the main goal you have just set yourself.

It doesn't really matter what the goal is, as long as you are ready to make some changes to achieve it. It may be a relatively small goal such as stopping drinking fruit juice. In this case, the change you need to make is quite obvious, and I would recommend that you ask yourself the questions on the previous page about how ready you are to make this change, to check it is achievable, and then to go for it. If you are successful this will spur you on to set yourself further challenges and goals.

It may be, however, that you set yourself quite a significant goal – such as no longer having hypos. In this case I would recommend that you break it down into specific changes that you feel you can make in order to ultimately achieve your goal – and to write them down. Alongside each one, write the scores to the two 'readiness to change' questions, and then add them up and put them in the final column. You will end up with something like this:

My goal is: ....

In order to do this I will aim to: ....

The Change	How important is it for me to do it? (0–10 scale)	How confident am I that I can do it? (0–10 scale)	Sum of both scores

I would suggest that right now, before going any further, you take some time to list the most realistic changes you can make to help you achieve your goal. If you need to read though some of the earlier chapters then do so, but please do it as soon as you can – and only read on once you have done so.

You will now have a table that looks something like this:

My goal is: *to stop having hypos*

In order to do this I will aim to:

Change	How important is it for me to do it? (0–10 scale)	How confident am I that I can do it? (0–10 scale)	Sum of both scores
Check my blood glucose before giving insulin	10	7	17
Count my carbs	8	6	14
Use a bolus advisor to ensure the correct dose	6	6	12
Avoid over correcting high glucose levels	8	8	16

In theory, the change with the highest score is the one that you will find easiest to do followed by the one with the next highest score. So, in this example the first thing to do will be to ensure you check your glucose level before injecting insulin. Now that is easier said than done, so what tricks can you employ to increase your chances of doing that? I sometimes use the acronym: T I E. Test – Inject – Eat, and encourage people to 'TIE' these actions together in the right order. Maybe writing that on the fridge door, or sticking a label on your insulin pen or vial, will help. Maybe getting someone close to you to remind you, gently, but not to nag as that will be counter-productive. Then you need to think about how you can achieve the other goals you have identified as being the most likely you can achieve, and when you will do so. It might be worth writing your answers down, as follows:

Change	How will I achieve this?	When will I start
Check my blood glucose before giving insulin	Write TIE in key places; get a second meter to keep at work	Today
Count my carbs	Use the carb counting app	next week
Use a bolus advisor to ensure the correct dose	Not sure	Not sure
Avoid over correcting high glucose levels	Reduce my correction dose	Now

Once you have achieved these changes then you can consider addressing the next item on your list and so on. You don't necessarily have to go through this process with every change you plan to make, but it may be helpful to start with. The aim is that you only plan to make changes that are SMART. That is:

Specific – so you know exactly what you are going to do;

Measurable – you know how to tell if you have achieved it;

Achievable – it has to be a change that you are able to make;

Realistic – and one which you have a realistic chance of making;

Timely – and one for which you can specify a time of making it.

Please note that the changes I have used in this example are just examples. You have to be honest in choosing the ones that are the SMARTest ones for you.

Having chosen your schedule of changes, allow yourself occasional treats and relax the rules on special occasions. Why? Because if you really don't like testing your glucose in certain situations when you are out, then you need to allow yourself not to in certain situations. You can minimise the risk by giving a low-carb meal and not injecting, but checking when you get home, or just giving a small dose, accepting your glucose might go high and commit to checking (and correcting if needed) when you get home.

Remember: you have developed your current eating and activity patterns over many years. Many of them will have become habits; behaviours that you follow because you always have done them. Some will be automatic – they are your 'default' way of behaving. It will not be easy to suddenly make a big change. As a general rule, therefore, you are more likely to achieve change in small steps; don't try to commit to too many changes all at once. Small changes to your diet (or activity levels that you feel you are able to maintain) are more likely to help you achieve your goal than a drastic change that you cannot stick to for more than a couple of weeks. Success with your first small changes will give you the confidence to embark on some of the more difficult changes on your list.

Eating is a social activity, and if you make changes to the what, when or how you eat, it will impact on others – especially those that you live with. So it helps to have others on board as you try to make changes. Maybe someone else in your household, or a close friend, could also do with making some changes to their diet or activity levels. If there is no one else who is willing or able to make changes with you, it will help if there is someone who you can confide in, and who can support you as you start your programme of making changes and encourage you to stick with them.

At the end of the day, the success you have will depend on your own motivation to make changes, and your ability to stick to them. Over time motivation may well diminish, and everyday life will get in the way. What may be the high priority today (making changes to control your diabetes) may be superseded by a friend or family member becoming unwell, or a financial problem or just about anything else that life can throw at us. It is completely natural that daily living and the many crises that occur take your focus away from lifestyle changes. Be aware that as a result, you may slip back into your previous eating habits, or to not checking glucose levels. If this does happen, please do not fall into the trap of blaming yourself or criticising yourself for failing.

Instead, focus on what you have achieved so far, and give yourself time to concentrate on the new priorities that have emerged in your life – without feelings of guilt. However, if possible, see what changes you are able to maintain during this period, and whether it is possible to set yourself a plan to restart the other changes in the near future. If not, perhaps you can commit to reviewing your progress in four weeks' time, for example, even if you then decide you cannot make any further progress right now. It may be that re-reading the goals you set yourself will help re-motivate you. As might speaking to a trusted friend, or someone on your diabetes team.

Having completed the goal-setting exercise above, it may be helpful to recap some of the key components to taking control of your diabetes, to ensure your goals cover all the main points and that your lifestyle changes are as effective as possible in controlling your glucose levels.

1. You may need to make changes to your diet. My recommendation is to adopt simple dietary changes as outlined in this book, which focus mainly on reducing sugars and starches (including sugar-sweetened drinks), and I know of many people who have used this approach to achieve much better control of their diabetes.

2. Would it help to discuss the changes you wish to make with a family member or a close friend? It may help to show them your goals and explain why and how you want to achieve them.

3. Are you confident that you are accurate in counting your carbohydrates? Would it be worth discussing whether there is a local session or course you can attend to update your skills?

4. Blood glucose monitoring is important in showing you how effective your lifestyle and insulin regimen are in controlling your glucose levels. Remember that ideally they should be between 4 and 6mmol/l (70–110mg/dl) before meals, and no higher than 8mmol/l (140mg/dl) after meals. Make sure you have an up-to-date meter (most pharmacies sell a selection) and that you use it according to the manufacturer's instructions. Consider whether you would benefit from one of the continuous monitoring systems now available, and whether you could afford to use this, if it is not covered by the NHS or your health plan.

5. Do you need to adjust your ICR or ISF? If you need help with this, is there someone in your diabetes team who can advise you?

6. Would you benefit from using an insulin pump? Is this something you would consider looking into?

7. Be realistic about what you can achieve. It likely took months and possibly years to develop your current method of managing your diabetes, so don't expect a miracle overnight. It is far better to

make steady changes that lead to gradual improvement over the course of weeks or months than to make drastic changes which you cannot keep up for longer than a few days.

Finally, I would like to thank you for taking the trouble to read this book. The aim of the book has been to help you identify how you can best take control of your diabetes, and to provide you with some advice on how to do it. While I and others can provide advice, only you can actually make the changes – good luck.

EPILOGUE

It is my hope that you will be able to use the information within this book to learn some techniques to help you better manage your diabetes in the months and years to come. If you live in the United Kingdom, then despite the challenges facing the National Health Service, you have reliable access to high-quality medical care, insulin and other medications, completely free of charge. If you live in another Western European country then there is good access to high-quality care, although with some charge that is generally affordable. The same applies in many other countries around the world.

When I left the comfort of the UK National Health Service to work for the International Diabetes Federation (IDF), I was shocked to learn that there are still too many countries where that is not the case. There are some rich countries where excellent care is available and yet some people cannot afford even basic necessities such as insulin or glucose test strips. I have experienced this first hand in recent work that I have done overseas.

There are also many poor countries where there is a shortage of diabetes specialists and sometimes even the basics are just not available. While I worked at the IDF, I helped coordinate a global survey that showed that basic human insulin was only available with any degree of certainty in 40 per cent of the poorest countries of the world. And when it was, it could cost up to two-thirds of a basic wage. Tragically, that means that in some countries, particularly in Africa, many children and young people die from type 1 diabetes, because of lack of insulin.

The United Nations has decreed that by 2030 every country should provide Universal Health Coverage to its citizens. That would mean that everyone with type 1 diabetes would receive at least basic care at an affordable cost. Even if that were to be achieved, then that still leaves countless people at risk of poor health or worse for many years to come, just because they cannot get the care they need.

There are a number of organisations that are trying to fill the gap in the meantime. The IDF's Life for a Child programme operates in 40 countries in all parts of the world. They work with local health services to provide good-quality healthcare and guarantee to provide insulin and supplies to young people with type 1 diabetes until the age of 25. $1 US a day (£0.70, €0.80) to help keep a young person with type 1 diabetes alive and well.

A proportion of the proceeds from sales of this book will be donated to Life for a Child. I know that we all have many competing demands on our finances and on our charitable giving, but if you benefit from free or affordable insulin, please consider doing something that will directly help a young person with type 1 diabetes receive the insulin and care that otherwise they could not afford.

Regular or one-off donations to Life for a Child can be made from any country in the world via www.lifeforachildusa.org
Thank you.

APPENDIX 1 - USEFUL WEBSITES

BERTIE TYPE 1 DIABETES EDUCATION PROGRAMME.

Originally developed by Dr David Cavan and Joan Everett in 2005, this online version of the BERTIE programme was fully updated in 2016 to provide useful information to help you to understand and manage your diabetes in a way that suits you and your lifestyle.

www.bertieonline.org.uk

BEYOND TYPE 1

A US site that aims to educate the global community about this chronic, autoimmune disease, as well as providing resources and support for those living with Type 1. Beyond Type 1 bridges the gap from diagnosis to cure, empowering people to both live well today and to fund a better tomorrow.

www.beyondtype1.org

CARBS & CALS

Carbs & Cals is a unique way of counting carbs, calories and other nutrients. Their products include books and apps and show thousands of photos of food portions, with the nutritional info shown for each photo.

www.carbsandcals.com

DIABETES.CO.UK

Diabetes.co.uk is a community website focusing on providing a comprehensive, supportive and independent experience for our visitors from across the world. Diabetes.co.uk has developed into Europe's largest community of people with diabetes and people without diabetes alike ...

www.diabetes.co.uk

DIABETES COMMUNITY

DiabetesCommunity.com is a global edition of the diabetes.co.uk website. It is a community of people with diabetes, their family members, friends, supporters and caretakers, all offering their own support, knowledge and first hand experiences.

www.diabetescommunity.com

DIABETES DAILY

Diabetes Daily is a US site that believes that everyone with diabetes can live a healthy, happy and hopeful life. Whether you are newly diagnosed, a fifty-year veteran, or supporting a loved one, they are there to help you thrive.

www.diabetesdaily.com

DIABETES SUPPORT FORUM UK

This site encourages people to share and discuss experiences, enabling them to better understand their condition, gain more control of it and work more effectively with their healthcare teams. It is genuinely independent, run by members, is non-commercial and is not affiliated to any organisation.

www.diabetes-support.org.uk

DIABETES TRAVEL

A US site for the diabetes community to provide information on the travel process with diabetes considerations in mind—what to pack, letters for travel, airport security, beach day advice and more!

www.diabetestravel.org

DIABETES UK

Diabetes UK is the leading UK charity for people affected by diabetes. Their vision is a world where diabetes can do no harm.

www.diabetes.org.uk

DIABETIC EYE SCREENING

Information about the UK eye screening service, regarded as one of the best systems in the world for the early detection of diabetic eye disease.

https://www.nhs.uk/Conditions/diabetic-eye-screening/

DIATHLETE

Set up by Gavin Griffiths, Diathlete aims to provide Type 1 diabetes education with encouragement. Their motto is Educate, Encourage, Empower

www.diathlete.org

EXCARBS

Excarbs is a US site whose aim is to help people with diabetes using insulin to feel comfortable with taking up exercise – the advice is not aimed at elite athletes but hopefully covers the basic rules for most people living with diabetes.

www.excarbs.com

INTERNATIONAL DIABETES FEDERATION

The global advocate for people with diabetes. The mission of IDF is to promote diabetes care, prevention and a cure worldwide.

www.idf.org

NHS CHOICES

Information from the National Health Service on diabetes, treatments, local services and healthy living.

www.nhs.uk/Conditions/Diabetes/Pages/Diabetes.aspx

PUBLIC LIBRARY OF SCIENCE

Non-profit organisation of scientists committed to making the world's scientific and medical literature freely accessible to scientists and to the public.

www.plos.org

RUNSWEET

A comprehensive site to support people with diabetes undertaking a wide range of different sports. The content of the site is by people with diabetes, who want to promote diabetes self care, and share knowledge on how to manage diabetes with different sports and exercises.

www.runsweet.com

T1 RESOURCES

T1 resources is a new UK site with useful links, websites and online communities that can help you manage type 1 diabetes.

www.t1resources.uk

APPENDIX 2 – CHARTS TO CHECK PUMP BASAL RATES

TO CHECK OVERNIGHT BASAL RATE

Eat a normal meal (ideally with less than 80g carbohydrate and without alcohol) by 8pm in the evening and then check your glucose levels at the following times. Have a normal breakfast at 8am:

Time	8pm	10	11	12	1am	2	3	4	5	6	7	8	9	10
Current basal rate														
Glucose level														
Grams carbohydrate														
Bolus dose														

TO CHECK MORNING BASAL RATE

Skip or have a carbohydrate-free breakfast at 8am and a normal lunch at 1pm. Check at the following times:

Time	8am	9	10	11	12	1pm	2	3
Current basal rate								
Glucose level								
Grams carbohydrate								
Bolus dose								

TO CHECK AFTERNOON BASAL RATE

Have a normal lunch at 1pm with no carbohydrate until 7pm. Then have a normal evening meal. Check at the following times:

Time	1pm	2	3	4	5	6	7	8	9
Current basal rate									
Glucose level									
Grams carbohydrate									
Bolus dose									

TO CHECK EVENING BASAL RATE

Have a normal evening meal at 6pm with no carbohydrate afterwards and check at the following times:

Time	6pm	7	8	9	10	11	12
Current basal rate							
Glucose level							
Grams carbohydrate							
Bolus dose							

Note that completing these charts will also enable you to check the bolus doses taken for breakfast, lunch and evening meals according to the time of day being assessed.

Glossary

A

ACE inhibitors
ACE inhibitors are a medication mainly used to lower blood pressure and the resulting strain on the heart. ACE stands for angiotensin converting enzyme. Angiotensin is a chemical that can make blood vessels narrower.

Albuminuria
Damaged kidneys may start to leak protein into the urine. Albumin is a small, abundant protein in the blood that passes through the kidney filter into the urine easier than other proteins. In people newly diagnosed with type 2 diabetes the kidneys may already show signs of small amounts of protein leakage called microalbuminuria. This may be because of diabetes or from other diseases seen in conjunction with diabetes such as high blood pressure. Protein in the urine increases the risk of developing end-stage kidney disease. It also means that the person is at a particularly high risk of the development of cardiovascular disease.

Alpha cells

Alpha cells are found in the islets of Langerhans in the pancreas. They produce and release glucagon.

Angiotensin II receptor antagonists

A class of drugs that work in a similar way to ACE inhibitors to reduce blood pressure. Angiotensin II receptor antagonists, also called angiotensin receptor blockers (ARBs), work by blocking the formation of angiotensin II, a substance that makes blood vessels narrower.

Antibodies

Proteins produced in the body that protect it from foreign substances such as bacteria or viruses. In auto-immune conditions, antibodies lead to destruction of healthy tissue. In the case of type 1 diabetes, these are the insulin-producing beta cells.

Artificial pancreas

A automated system that comprises a continuous glucose sensor and an insulin pump. The infusion rate of the pump is determined by the glucose level measured by the sensor.

B

Basal insulin

Also termed, 'background insulin', the basal insulin is designed to keep the blood glucose stable overnight and between meals. It is provided by one or two injections of intermediate or long-acting insulin, or by a continuous infusion (via an insulin pump) of rapid or short-acting insulin.

Beta cells

Beta cells are found in the islets of Langerhans in the pancreas. They produce and release insulin type 1 diabetes, they are destroyed by the immune system.

Blood glucose meter

A meter that measures the concentration of glucose in a blood sample applied to the end of a test strip, inserted into the meter. Some meters incorporate bolus advisors to calculate the required insulin dose, based on the measured glucose level.

Blood pressure

Blood pressure is the amount of force that is exerted by blood on the blood vessels. It is measured in millimetres of mercury (written as mm Hg). When blood pressure is taken the measurement is given as two numbers, for example 120/80 mm Hg. The first number is called the systolic pressure and is the measure of pressure in the arteries when the heart beats and pushes more blood into the arteries. The second number, called the diastolic pressure, is the pressure in the arteries when the heart rests between beats. The ideal blood pressure for non-pregnant people with diabetes is 130/80 or less.

Bolus insulin

Also known as mealtime insulin. An injection of short-acting or rapid-acting insulin given just prior to a meal. The dose is calculated using the insulin to carbohydrate ratio and the insulin sensitivity factor.

C

Carbohydrate

A carbohydrate is a large organic molecule consisting of carbon (C), hydrogen (H) and oxygen (O) atoms. The term is most common in biochemistry, where it is synonymous with saccharide (sugar). The lighter versions of the molecules (monosaccharides and disaccharides) are commonly referred to as sugars. Carbohydrates perform numerous roles in living organisms including the storage of energy (e.g. starch and glycogen) and in an informal context, the term carbohydrate often means any food that is particularly rich in the complex carbohydrate starch (such as cereals, bread, and pasta) or simple carbohydrates such as table sugar.

Carbohydrate counting

The system by which a person with diabetes is able to estimate the amount of carbohydrate (usually expressed as grams of carbohydrate) in their meals. The insulin to carbohydrate ratio is then used to convert this into the required insulin dose for each meal.

Cardiovascular disease (CVD)

Cardiovascular diseases are defined as diseases that and injuries of the circulatory system: the heart, the blood vessels of the heart and the system of blood vessels throughout the body ad to (and in) the brain. Stroke is the result of a blood flow problem within, or leading to, the brain and is considered a form of CVD.

Cholesterol

A waxy substance made by the liver that is an essential part of cell walls and nerves. Cholesterol plays an important role in body functions such as digestion and hormone production. In addition to being produced by the body cholesterol comes from foods that we eat. Too much cholesterol in the blood causes an increase in particles called LDL ('bad' cholesterol), which increases the build up of plaque in the artery walls and leads to atherosclerosis.

Continuous glucose monitoring (CGM)

The use of a sensor inserted beneath the skin that measures the concentration of glucose in the fat below the skin, to provide a continuous reading of the glucose level. The level is not exactly the same as the level in the blood, but provides an accurate estimation of the blood glucose. Some CGM systems are connected to an insulin pump and can automatically stop the insulin infusion of the measured glucose level is too low.

D

Dawn phenomenon

This described the tendency for the blood glucose level to rise in the early hours of the morning as a result of the effect of hormones such as growth hormone and cortisol which are at the highest at these times. If it causes a marked increase in glucose, it is best managed by use of an insulin pump.

Diabetes complications

Diabetes complications are acute and chronic conditions caused by diabetes. Chronic complications include retinopathy (eye disease), nephropathy (kidney disease), neuropathy (nerve disease), cardiovascular disease (disease of the circulatory system), foot ulceration and amputation.

Diabetes mellitus (DM)

Diabetes mellitus is a chronic condition that arises when the pancreas does not produce enough insulin or when the body cannot effectively use the insulin produced. There are two basic forms of diabetes: type 1 and type 2. People with type 1 diabetes do not produce any insulin. People with type 2 diabetes produce insulin but cannot use it effectively.

Diabetes distress

The emotional and psychological burden experienced by people with diabetes. It can be caused by fear of hypoglycaemia, or fear of complications for example. It can cause anxiety and is associated with high HbA1c.

Diabetic foot

A foot that exhibits any pathology that results directly from diabetes or complications of diabetes.

Diabetic ketoacidosis (DKA)

DKA happens when there is not enough insulin and cells are unable to use glucose for energy. An alternative source of energy called ketones becomes activated. The system creates a build up of acids and can lead to coma and even death.

E

Epidemiology

The study of the occurrence and distribution of health-related states or events in specific populations, including the study of the determinants influencing such states, and the applications of this knowledge to the control of health problems.

F

Fats

Substances that help the body utilise some vitamins and help keep the skin healthy. They are also the main way the body stores energy. In food, there are many types of fats: saturated, unsaturated, polyunsaturated, monounsaturated and trans fats.

Flash Glucose Monitoring

A term coined to describe the type of monitoring provided by systems such as the Freestyle Libre, in which a glucose sensor is inserted below the skin and provides a reading when a reading device is passed over it. This is in contrast to continuous glucose monitoring systems which provide a continuous display of glucose levels.

Fructose

A type of sugar found in many fruits and vegetables and in honey.

G

Gestational diabetes mellitus (GDM)

Diabetes first diagnosed during pregnancy.

Glucagon

A hormone secreted by the pancreas; stimulates increases in blood sugar levels in the blood (thus opposing the action of insulin).

Glucose

Also called dextrose. The main sugar the body produces from proteins, fats and carbohydrates. Glucose is the major source of energy for living cells. However, the cells cannot use glucose without the help of insulin.

Glycemic index (GI)

Glycemic index is a measure of how quickly blood glucose rise after eating a particular type of food. Glucose has a glycemic index of 100. The effects that different foods have on blood glucose levels vary considerably. The glycemic index estimates how much each gram of available carbohydrate (total carbohydrate minus fiber) in a food raises a person's blood glucose level following consumption of the food, relative to consumption of pure glucose.

Glycogen

Glycogen is a long molecule of linked-together glucose units (polysaccharide) that acts as a form of energy storage in animals. This polysaccharide structure represents the main storage form of glucose in the body and is analogous to starch, the energy storage molecule found in plants.

In humans, glycogen is made and stored primarily in the cells of the liver and the muscles, and functions as the secondary long-term energy storage. Muscle glycogen is converted into glucose by muscle cells, and liver glycogen converts to glucose for use throughout the body. As an energy reserve, it can be quickly drawn upon to meet a sudden need for glucose.

Glycosylated haemoglobin (HbA1c)

See below

H

HbA1c (glycated hemoglobin)

Haemoglobin is a protein in red blood cells that comprises of globin and iron-containing haem, which transports oxygen from the lungs to the tissues of the body. Glycosylated haemoglobin is haemoglobin to which glucose is chemically bound. It is tested to monitor long-term control of diabetes. The level of glycosylated haemoglobin is increased in the red blood cells of persons with poorly controlled diabetes.

Honeymoon period

A period, usually in the first two years following diagnosis of type 1 diabetes, when some insulin is still produced by the pancreas. During a honeymoon period, people can manage with very low insulin doses.

Hormone

A chemical substance secreted by an endocrine gland or group of endocrine cells that acts to control or regulate specific physiological processes, including growth, metabolism, and reproduction. Most hormones are secreted by endocrine cells in one part of the body and then transported by the blood to their target site of action in another part, though some hormones act only in the region in which they are secreted

Hyperglycaemia

A raised level of glucose in the blood, a sign that diabetes is out of control. It occurs when the body does not have enough insulin or cannot use the insulin it does have to turn glucose into energy. Signs of hyperglycaemia are of great thirst, dry mouth and a need to urinate often.

Hypertension

Abnormally high blood pressure, especially in the arteries. Often referred to as high blood pressure. High blood pressure increases the risk for heart attack and stroke.

Hypoglycaemia

Too low a level of glucose in the blood. This occurs when a person with diabetes has injected too much insulin, eaten too little food or has exercised without extra food. A person with hypoglycaemia may feel nervous, shaky, weak, sweaty and have a headache, blurred vision and hunger.

I

Impaired fasting glucose (IFG)

Impaired fasting glucose (IFG) is a category of higher than normal blood glucose, but below the diagnostic threshold for diabetes after fasting (typically after an overnight fast). People with IFG are at an increased risk of developing diabetes.

Impaired glucose tolerance (IGT)

Impaired glucose tolerance (IGT) is a category of higher than normal blood glucose but below the diagnostic threshold for diabetes, after ingesting a standard amount of glucose in an oral glucose tolerance test. People with IGT are at an increased risk of developing diabetes.

Immune therapy

Treatment that is aimed at modifying the immune attack on the beta cells to halt the development of type 1 diabetes. Many clinical trials have explored such treatments, ususally at the time of diagnosis but to date none has been successful in preventing the onset of type 1 diabetes

Incidence

It indicates how often a disease occurs. More precisely, it corresponds to the number of new cases of a disease among certain groups if people for a certain period of time.

Impotence

Also called erectile dysfunction and is a persistent inability of the penis to become erect or stay erect. Some men may become impotent after having diabetes for a long time because nerves and blood vessels in the penis become damaged.

Insulin

A hormone whose main action is to enable the body cells to absorb glucose from the blood and use it as energy. Insulin is produced by the beta cells of the islets of Langerhans in the pancreas. People with type 1 diabetes need regular insulin injections to stay alive.

Insulin analogues

Preparations of insulin in which the insulin molecule has been modified in order to speed up (in the case of rapid-acting analogues) or slow down (long-acting analogues) its absorption.

Insulin resistance

Insulin resistance (IR) is the condition in which cells fail to respond to the normal actions of the hormone insulin. It is usually seen in people who are overweight, or who have prediabetes or type 2 diabetes. The body produces insulin, but the cells in the body become resistant to insulin and are unable to use it as effectively, leading to hyperglycemia. Beta cells in the pancreas subsequently increase their production of insulin.

Insulin sensitivity factor (ISF)

The effect of one unit of insulin in reducing the glucose level in the blood. The ISF is used to calculate a correction dose for when the glucose level is too high.

Insulin pump

A wearable device that contains a reservoir of insulin that is infused through a cannula into the subcutaneous tissue. It provides a continuous basal infusion of insulin that can be programmed to change at different times of the day.

Insulin to carbohydrate ratio (ICR)

This can be expressed as the amount of insulin required to be given for each 10 grams of carbohydrate in a meal (eg 1.5 units per 10g); or as the number of grams of carbohydrate that require one unit of insulin (eg 7g for 1 unit). It is used to calculate the amount of insulin to be injected for meals containing carbohydrate.

Islets of Langerhans

Named after the German anatomist, Paul Langerhan, who discovered them in 1869, these clusters of cells are located in the pancreas and contain its endocrine (hormone-producing) cells. They make up approximately 2 per cent of the pancreas.

N

Nephropathy

Caused by the damage to small blood vessels and cause the kidneys to become less efficient or fail altogether.

Neuropathy

Occurs when blood glucose and blood pressure are too high, diabetes can harm nerves throughout the body and cause damage to the nerves.

The pancreas

The pancreas is a glandular organ situated behind the lower part of the stomach and contains endocrine cells that produce the critical hormones insulin and glucagon and also has a digestive role.

O

Obesity

The term used to describe excess body fat. It is defined in terms of an individual's weight and height or his/her body mass index (BMI). A BMI over 30 is classified as being obese. Obesity makes your body less sensitive to insulin's action and extra body fat is thought to be a risk factor for diabetes.

P

Protein

Proteins are one of three main types of food and are made of amino acids, which are called the building blocks of the cells. All cells need protein to grow and to repair themselves. Protein is found in many foods such as meat, fish, poultry, eggs, legumes, and dairy products.

R

Randomised controlled trials

These are trials designed to test whether a treatment is effective. Participants are split into groups. One group is given the treatment being tested while another group (called the comparison or control group) is given an alternative treatment, which could be a different type of drug or a dummy treatment (a placebo). The results are then compared.

Renal

Relating to the kidneys.

Retina

Part of the back lining of the eye that senses light and is fed by many small blood vessels that can be damaged by diabetes.

Retinopathy

Retinopathy is a disease of the retina of the eye, which may cause visual impairment or blindness.

S

Somogyi effect

Describes the phenomenon whereby the blood glucose level rises following a hypoglycaemic attack, typically but not always during the night, thought to be due to the effect of adrenalin and other hormones released as a result of the hypo.. It was first reported in the 1930s but more recent researchers doubt its existence. Many people with type 1 diabetes recognise its occurrence.

Starch

Starch is a carbohydrate consisting of a large number of glucose units joined together. A polysaccharide, it is produced by most green plants as an energy store. It is the most common carbohydrate in human diets and is contained in large amounts in such staple foods as potatoes, wheat, maize (corn) and rice.

Stroke

A sudden loss of function in part of the blain as a result of the interruption of its blood supply by a blocked or burst artery.

T

Triglyceride

Fats carried in the blood and derived from the foods we eat. Most of the fats we eat, including butter, margarines, and oils, are in triglyceride form. An excess of triglycerides are stored in fat cells throughout the body. The body needs insulin to remove this type of fat from the blood.

Type 1 diabetes

Type 1 diabetes mellitus develops most frequently in children and adolescents. About 10 per cent of people with diabetes have type 1. The symptoms of type 1 vary in intensity and include excessive thirst, excessive passing of urine, weight loss and lack of energy. Insulin is a life-sustaining medication for people with type 1 diabetes and they require daily injections for survival.

Type 2 diabetes

Type 2 diabetes mellitus is much more common than type 1 and occurs mainly in adults, although it is now seen increasingly in children and adolescents. The symptoms of type 1 may affect people with type 2 but to a lesser degree. Some people with type 2, however, have no early symptoms and are only diagnosed several years after the onset of the condition when various diabetic complications are already present. Recent scientific research has shown that fat deposited in the liver and pancreas may be impairing the functions of these organs and causing type 2 diabetes. Reversal (partial or complete) of the condition is now thought possible through a combination of calorie restriction and increased physical activity.

REFERENCE NOTES

1. Rollo J. Diabetes mellitus: an account of two cases of diabetes mellitus: with remarks as they arose during the progress of the cure. Ann Med 1797; 85–106.
2. von Mering J, Minkowski O. Diabetes mellitus nach Pankreas extirpation. Arch f exper Path u Pharmakol. 1889; 26:371.
3. Banting FG, et al. The Effect Produced on Diabetes by Extractions of Pancreas. Transact Ass Amer Physicians. 1922; 37:337.
4. Pociot F, Lernmark A. Genetic risk factors for type 1 diabetes. Lancet 2016; 387; 2231–2339.
5. Rewers M, Ludvigsson J. Environmental risk factors for type 1 diabetes. Lancet 2016; 387: 2340–2348.
6. Knip M, et al. Hydrolyzed Infant Formula and Early β-Cell Autoimmunity: A Randomized Clinical Trial. JAMA. 2014; 311: 2279–2287.
7. Mohr SB, et al. The association between ultraviolet B irradiance, vitamin D status and incidence rates of type 1 diabetes in 51 regions worldwide. Diabetologia 2008; 51:1391–1398.
8. Zipitis CS, et al. Vitamin D supplementation in early childhood and risk of type 1 diabetes: a systematic review and meta-analysis. Arch Dis Child 2008; 93:512–517.
9. Scheiner G. *Think Like a Pancreas*. Da Capo Lifelong Books, Cambridge, Massachusetts 2012.
10. National Institute for Health and Care Excellence. Type 1 diabetes in adults: diagnosis and management. www.nice.org.uk/guidance/ng17

11. The Eatwell Guide. Public Health England, 2015. www.gov.uk/government/publications/the-eatwell-guide

12. Evidence-based nutrition guidelines for the prevention and management of diabetes. Diabetes UK 2018.

13. BERTIEonline: www.bertieonline.org.uk

14. Misra S, Oliver N. Diabetic ketoacidosis in adults. BMJ 2015; 351:h5660.

15. Naik S. Addressing the educational and psychological issues in type 1 diabetes. University of Southampton PhD thesis, Southampton 2010.

16. Eight tips for healthy eating. Live Well – NHS Choices. www.nhs.uk/Livewell/Goodfood/Pages/eight-tips-healthy-eating.aspx

17. Basu, S, et al., The relationship of sugar to population-level diabetes prevalence: an econometric analysis of repeated cross sectional data. PLoS ONE, 8, (2013), e57873, doi:10.1371/journal.pone.0057873

18. Lustig, RH. Fructose: metabolic, hedonic, and societal parallels with ethanol. Journal of the American Dietetic Association 2010 110:1307–21.

19. NHS choices, 5 a day: what counts? ww.nhs.uk/Livewell/5ADAY/Pages/Whatcounts.aspx

20. Is your fruit smoothie as healthy as you think? *Which?*, Dec 2012. www.which.co.uk/news/2012/12

21. *Carbs & Cals*. www.carbsandcals.com

22. Daley Kinsey, Diabetes daily. www.diabetesdaily.com/blog/the-five-stages-of-grieving-diabetes-165860

23. Naik S. Addressing the educational and psychological issues in type 1 diabetes. University of Southampton PhD thesis, Southampton 2010.

24. Bober E, et al. Partial remission phase and metabolic control in type 1 diabetes mellitus in children and adolescents. J Pediatr Endocrinol Metab. 2001; 14: 435–41.

25. Lean MEJ, et al. Dietary recommendations for people with diabetes: an update for the 1990s. Journal of human nutrition and dietetics 1991; 4:393–412.

26. Somogyi M. Insulin as a cause of extreme hyperglycaemia and instability. Bull St Louis Med Soc. 1938; 32: 498–500.

27. Hibbert-Jones E. Fat and protein counting in type 1 diabetes. Practical Diabetes 2016; 33: 243–247.

28. Peters AL, Davidson MB. Protein and fat effects on glucose responses and insulin requirements in subjects with insulin-dependent diabetes mellitus. Am J Clin Nutr 1993; 58: 555–60.

29. Paterson MA, et al. Influence of dietary protein on postprandial blood glucose levels in individuals with Type 1 diabetes mellitus using intensive insulin therapy. Diabet Med 2016; 33: 592–598.

30. Shula AP, et al. Food order has a significant impact on postprandial glucose.

31. Pankowska E, et al. Does the fat-protein meal increase postprandial glucose level in type 1 diabetes patients on insulin pump? The conclusion of a randomised study. Diabetes Technol Ther 2012; 14: 16–22.

32. Bao J, et al. Improving the estimation of mealtime insulin doses in adults with type 1 diabetes: the Normal Insulin Demand for Dose Adjustment (NIDDA) study. Diabetes Care 2011; 34: 146–51.

33. Ziegler R, et al. Use of an insulin bolus advisor improves glycemic control in multiple daily insulin injection (MDI) therapy patients with suboptimal glycemic control. Diabetes Care 2013; 36:3613–3619.

34. Oriot P, et al. Can an electronic glycaemic notebook associated with an insulin calculator improve HbA1c in diabetic patients on a multiple insulin injections regimen? A 26-week observational real-life study. Acta Clin Belg 2016; 71: 51–6.

35. Van Niel J, et al. Use of a smart glucose monitoring system to guide insulin dosing in patients with diabetes in regular clinical practice. J Diabetes sci Technol 2014; 8: 188–189.

36. Public Health Collaboration. Healthy eating guidelines and weight-loss advice for the UK, 2017 <https://phcuk.org/wp-content/uploads/2016/05/Healthy-Eating-Guidelines-Weight-Loss-Advice-For-The-United-Kingdom-Public-Health-Collaboration.pdf>

37. Lawrence RD. *The Diabetic ABC: A Practical Guide for Patients and Nurses*. London, HK Lewis 1964.

38. Nielsen JV, et al. Low carbohydrate diet in type 1 diabetes, long-term improvement and adherence: a clinical audit. Diabetology and Metabolic Syndrome 2012; 4: 23–27.

39. Krebs JD, et al. A randomised trial of the feasibility of a low carbohydrate diet vs standard carbohydrate counting in adults with type 1 diabetes taking body weight into account. Asia Pac J Clin Natr 2016; 25: 78–84.

40. Bernstein RK. *Dr Bernstein's Diabetes Solution*. Little, Brown and Company, Boston 2011.

41. www.type1keto.com

42. Lean mass hyper-responders. www.cholesterolcode.com/are-you-a-lean-mass-hyper-responder/

43. Pozzilli P. et al. Continuous subcutaneous insulin infusion in diabetes: patient populations, safety, efficacy and pharmacoeconomics. Diabetes Metab Research and reviews. 2016; 32: 21-39.19

44. Jenkins E, et al. Preparation for pumps: what difference could it make? Diabetic Med 2011; 28 (supp 1).

45. Jenkins E, et al. Improving the outcomes of pump therapy. Diabetis Med 2012; 29 (supp 1): 10.

46. Bode B, et al. Comparison of insulin aspart with buffered regular insulin and insulin lispro in continuous subcutaneous insulin infusion: a randomised study in type 1 diabetes. Diabetes Care 2002; 25: 439–444.

47. The Juvenile Diabetes Research Foundation Continuous Glucose Monitoring Study Group. Continuous glucose monitoring and intensive treatment of type 1 diabetes. New Eng J Med 2008; 359: 1464–76.

48. Foster NC, et al. Continuous glucose monitoring in patients with type 1 diabetes using insulin injections. Diabetes Care 2016; 39: e81–e82.

49. Lind M, et al. Continuous glucose monitoring vs conventional therapy for glycemic control in adults with type 1 diabetes treated with multiple daily injections. The GOLD randomised clinical trial. JAMA 2017; 317: 379–387.

50. Bolinder J et al. Novel glucose-sensing technology and hypoglycaemia in type 1 diabetes: a multicentre, non-masked, randomised controlled trial. Lancet 2016; 388: 2254–2263.

51. Danne T, et al. Prevention of hypoglycaemia using low glucose suspend function in sensor-augmented pump therapy. Diabetes Technol Ther 2011; 13: 1129–1134.

52. Pastor A, et al. Alcohol and recreational drug use in young adults with type 1 diabetes. Diabetes Res Clin Practice 2017; 130: 186–195.

53. Turner BC, et al. The effect of evening alcohol consumption on next-morning glucose control in type 1 diabetes. Diabetes Care 2001; 24: 1888–93.

54. Ismail D, et al. Social consumption of alcohol in adolescents with type 1 diabetes is associated with increased glucose lability, but not hypoglycaemia. Diab Med 2006; 23: 830–3.

55. Ng RS, et al. Street drug use among young patients with type 1 diabetes in the UK. Diabetic Med 2004; 21: 295–6.

56. ExCarbs, at www.diabetesnet.com/diabetes-control/exercise-and-diabetes/excarbs-exercise

57. Bussau V, et al. The 10-s maximal sprint. Diabetes Care 2006; 29: 601–606.

58. Iscoe KE, Riddell MC. Continuous moderate-intensity exercise with or without intermittent high-intensity work: effects on acute and late glycaemia in athletes with type 1 diabetes mellitus. Diabet Med 2011; 28: 824–832.

59. www.thenoakesfoundation.org/nutrition-network/the-lchf-diet-for-elite-athletes-in-high-intensity-sport

60. www.runsweet.com

61. www.diathlete.org

62. Lets talk about sex, at Beyond Type 1. www.beyondtype1.org/lets-talk-about-sex

63. National Institute for Health and Care Excellence. Diabetes in pregnancy: management from preconception to the postnatal period. 2015, nice.org.uk/guidance/ng3

64. Guerin A, et al. Use of maternal GHb concentration to estimate the risk of congenital anomalies in the offspring of women with prepregnancy diabetes. Diabetes Care. 2007; 30:1920–5.

65. Asbjornsdottir B, et al. The influence of carbohydrate consumption on glycaemic control in pregnant women with type 1 diabetes. Diab Res Clin Pract 2017; 127: 97–104.

66. Das A, et al. New treatments for diabetic retinopathy. Diabetes, Obesity and Metabolism 2014; 17: 219–230.

67. Estruch R, et al. Primary prevention of cardiovascular disease with a Mediterranean diet. New Eng J Med 2013; 368: 1279–1290.

68. Shaban MC, et al. The prevalence of depression and anxiety in adults with type 1 diabetes. Diabet Med 2006; 23: 1381–4.

69. Shaban MC, et al. The relationship between generic and diabetes specific psychological factors and glycaemic control in adults with type 1 diabetes. Diabetes Res Clin Pract 2009; 85: e26–9.

70. Reddy J, et al. Putting PAID to diabetes-related distress: the potential utility of the problem areas in diabetes (PAID) scale in patinets with diabetes. Psychosomatics 2013; 54: 44–51.

71. The DAWN study. www.dawnstudy.com/DAWN2/dawn2.asp

72. Nimri R, et al. MD-Logic overnight control for 6 weeks of home use in patients with type 1 diabetes: randomised crossover trial. Diabetes Care 2014; 37: 3025–3032.

73. Kropff J, et al. Two month evening and night closed-loop glucose control in patients with type 1 diabetes under free-living conditions: a randomised crossover trial. Lancet Diabetes Endocrinol 2015; 3: 939–947.

74. Thabit H, et al. Home use of an artificial beta cell in type 1 diabetes. N Engl J Med 2015; 373: 2129–40.

75. FDA approves first automated insulin delivery. www.fda.gov/NewsEvents/Newsroom/PressAnnouncements/ucm522974.htm

76. van Bon AC, et al. Feasibility of a portable bihormonal closed loop system to control glucose excursions at home under freeliving conditions for 48 hours. Diabetes Technol Ther 2014; 16: 131–136.

77. Shapiro AMJ, et al. Islet transplantation in seven patients with type 1 diabetes mellitus using a glucocorticoid-free immunosuppressive regimen. *N Engl J Med* 2000; 343: 230–8.

78. Pagliuca FW, et al. Generation of functional human pancreatic β-cells in vitro. Cell 2014: http://dx.doi.org/10.1016/j.cell.2014.09.040

79. Rezania A, et al. Reversal of diabetes with insulin-producing cells derived in vitro from human pluripotent stem cells. Nature biotechnology 2014; 32: 1121–1133.

80. Haahr MK, et al. Safety and potential effect of a single intracavernous injection of autologous adipose-derived regenerative cells in patients with erectile dysfunction following radical prostatectomy: an open-label phase 1 clinical trial. EbioMedicine 2016; 5: 204–210.

81. Sharples EJ, et al. Challenges in pancreas transplantation. Acta Diabetol 2016; 53: 871–878.

82. Faustman DL, et al. Proof-of-Concept, Randomized, Controlled Clinical Trial of Bacillus-Calmette-Guerin for Treatment of Long-Term Type 1 Diabetes. PLoS ONE 7(8):e41756. doi:10.1371/journal.pone.0041756.

83. Cheng C, et al. Fasting-Mimicking Diet Promotes Ngn3-Driven β-Cell Regeneration to Reverse Diabetes. Cell 2017; e12: 775–788.

84. Toth C, et al. Type 1 diabetes mellitus successfully managed with the paleolithic ketogenic diet. Int J Case Rep Images 2014; 5: 699–703.

ACKNOWLEDGEMENTS

First and foremost, I wish to acknowledge the contribution of the thousands of people with type 1 diabetes who over many years have taught me so much about the complexities and challenges of living with type 1 diabetes, day in, day out. Special thanks are due to those who granted permission for me to describe aspects of their story.

I am also hugely indebted to the talented team at the Bournemouth Diabetes and Endocrine Centre, with whom I had the privilege of working for so many years, and who were always willing to try out new ideas in the quest to help people better manage their type 1 diabetes. I am particularly grateful to Joan Everett and Emma Jenkins who were pivotal in supporting the early work that led to the development of the BERTIE programme. Thanks to them, and also to Clare Shaban, Melanie Weiss and Jacky Ryder who kindly reviewed parts of the manuscript. Thanks also to Dr Sarita Naik who gave permission for me to cite much of her research work conducted in the department, and to Chris Cheyette who prepared the table on carbohydrate portion sizes. I am very grateful to Paul Warren, Ian Lake, Matthew Balch, Daniel Vegh and Emma Porter for reviewing the manuscript from a 'user's' viewpoint. The contributions of others are acknowledged in the text. I am indebted to my literary agent Jonathan Hayden and to my publisher Penguin Random House for their support in the writing and publishing of the book.

Finally, I wish to acknowledge the contribution of my wife Mary, both for her constant and ongoing support as I wrote this book, and also for all that I have learnt from her about overcoming the constant uncertainties and anxieties that come with living with an incurable long-term condition; I hope that these experiences have made me more understanding of the needs of people with type 1 diabetes and their loved ones.

INDEX

Page references in *italics* indicate tables and illustrations.

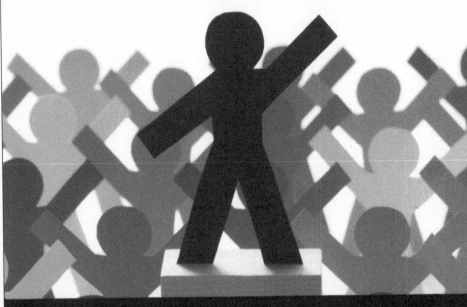
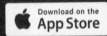 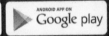
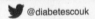 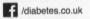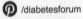